"Mitch Tonks is a legend, he makes simple, delicious food that I want to eat."
Jamie Oliver

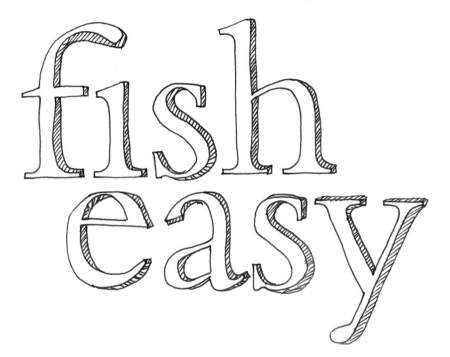

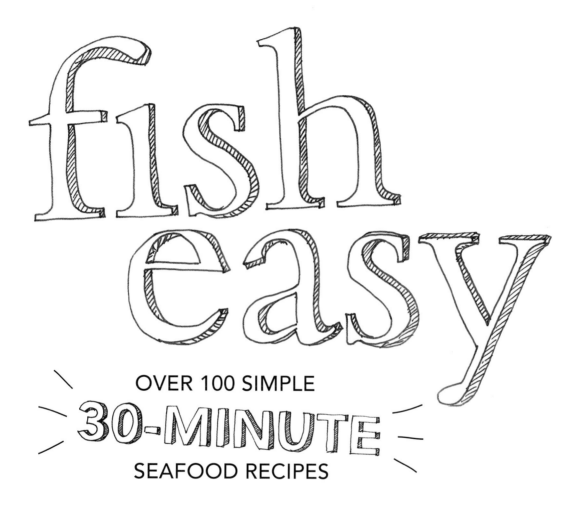

fish easy

OVER 100 SIMPLE **30-MINUTE** SEAFOOD RECIPES

MITCH TONKS

PAVILION

For Adam

This book is dedicated to the memory of my best friend
Adam Reynolds, one of the greatest people I ever had
the pleasure of knowing.

First published in the United Kingdom in 2012 by
PAVILION BOOKS
10 Southcombe Street
London
W14 0RA

An imprint of Anova Books Company Ltd

 Supported by Norwegian Seafood

Commissioning editor: Becca Spry
Design concept and cover: Georgina Hewitt
Layout: Miranda Harvey
Photographer: Chris Terry
Stylist: Cynthia Inions
Home economist: Sonja Edridge
Copy editor: Barbara Dixon
Production: Laura Brodie
Proofreader: Maggie Ramsay
Indexer: Hilary Bird

ISBN: 978-1-86205-929-0

A CIP catalogue record for this book is available from the British Library.
10 9 8 7 6 5 4 3 2 1
Colour reproduction by Rival Colour Ltd, UK
Printed and bound by Toppan Leefung Printing Ltd, China

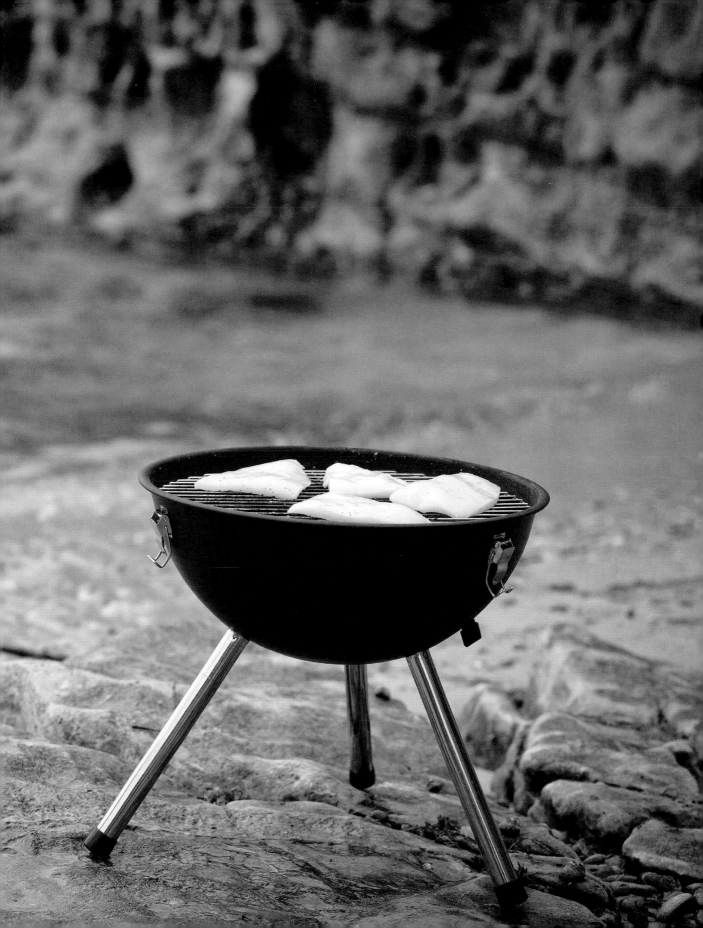

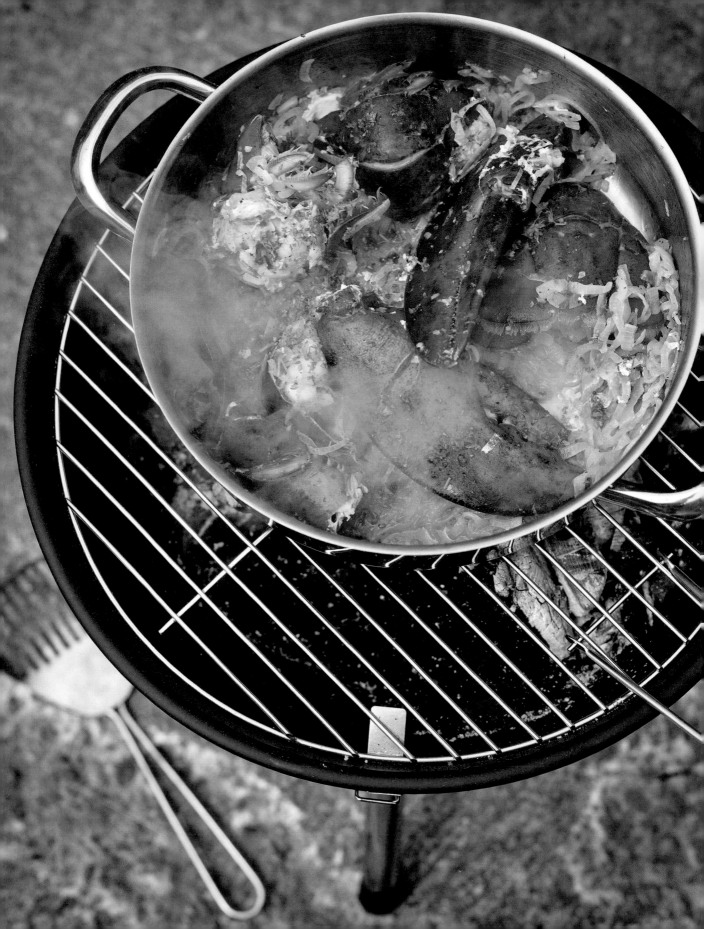

contents

introduction 8

on the grill 14

in the pan 58

in the oven 98

raw, cured and salads 150

mayonnaise and other basics 192

index 212

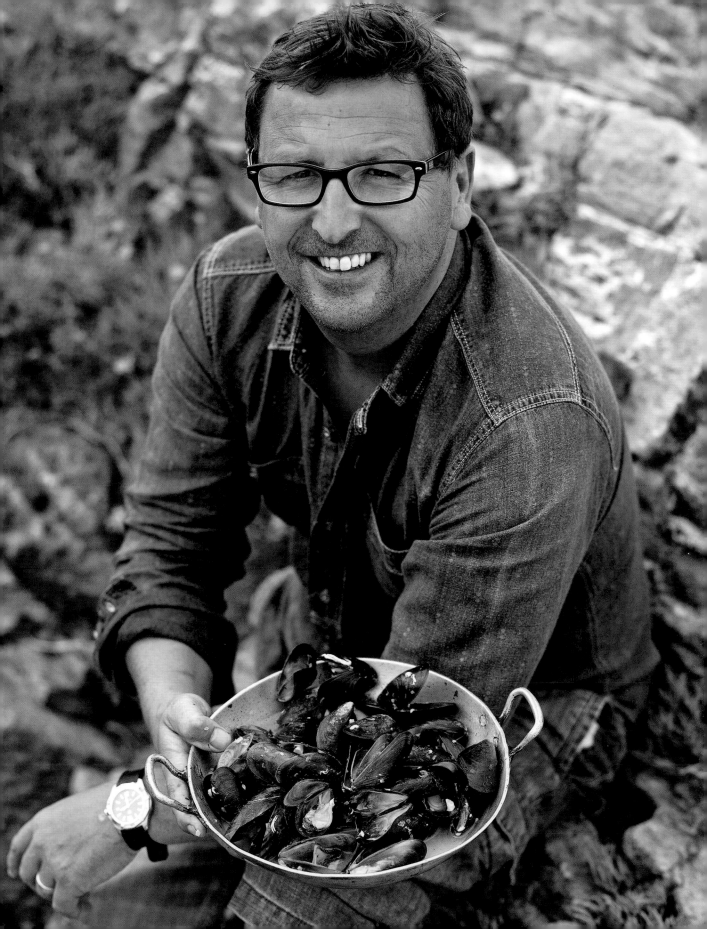

introduction

I am a self-taught cook who has learnt my trade from a handful of great books, my travels and my palate. I discovered many years ago that the most enjoyable fish dishes were the local specialities in any given place, for example bouillabaisse in southern France, *fritto misto* in Italy and lobster *caldereta* in the north of Menorca. I also found that the very simple preparation of anything fresh, from a grilled sole to a fish roasted with a few herbs, pleased me greatly. Successful seafood cookery relies upon two things – freshness and simple preparation – it's as uncomplicated as that.

Supply is often an issue; the number of independent fishmongers is declining and we are left mainly with the supermarket counter to buy from. Of course, having been a fishmonger I would always advocate finding a good one near to you and supporting him, but the supermarket is perfectly acceptable.

Frozen seafood is also a good alternative to fresh. Much of the fish that you buy from the chilled counter in the supermarket will have been frozen anyway; it's convenient if you wish to eat it on the day you buy it – but don't refreeze it.

Unlike meat, most fish is fine if cooked from frozen – which makes it the ultimate fast food. A frozen piece of fish cooked in a bag in the oven can produce excellent results with just a few added flavours. If we are to eat seafood sustainably, the acceptance of frozen seafood is a must, as much of it will have been fished from areas where stocks are well managed and fishing methods selective. When fish is caught a long way from land or distribution, to ship or fly it in fresh would make no sense, not least because complicated logistics put the product at risk of spoilage.

The provenance of seafood is as important as its freshness, and we should be buying fish from sustainable sources. Any species that has MSC (Marine Stewardship Council) certification will give you this surety, as should buying from local fishermen if you live near the coast. Naturally we are all concerned about the pressure commercial fishing puts on fish stocks, but we can still safely enjoy a wide variety of species as fisheries around the world adapt to the science of marine management. The cod and haddock fisheries in Norway are an example of what can be achieved when fishermen and scientists work together. The fisheries there produce some of the highest quality fish I have seen and they currently have the benefit of MSC certification.

This book will guide you through some straightforward cooking techniques based around the oven, the frying pan, the grill and the barbecue. There are also recipes for cured and raw fish. All the dishes are really simple to make – just choose one that appeals and off you go.

When it comes to marrying flavours with fish, the simple rule is – not too many flavours. Fish is great with sauces or salads that are a little acidic or piquant, made with ingredients such as capers, lemon, sorrel, limes, gherkins and mayonnaise. You will soon get the feel for flavouring and be creating your own combinations. These recipes make a great starting point.

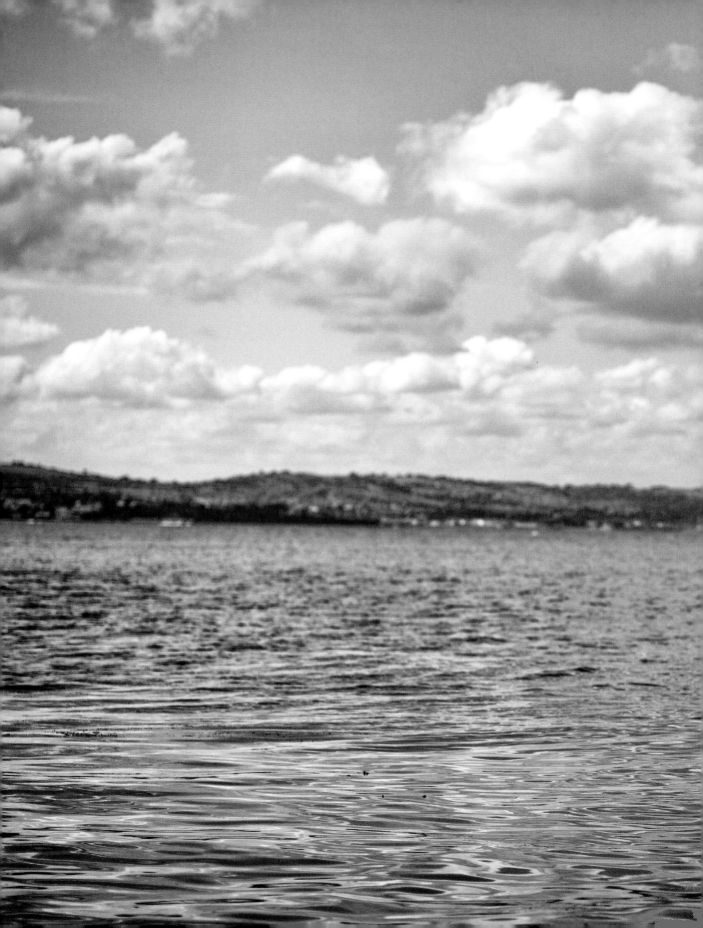

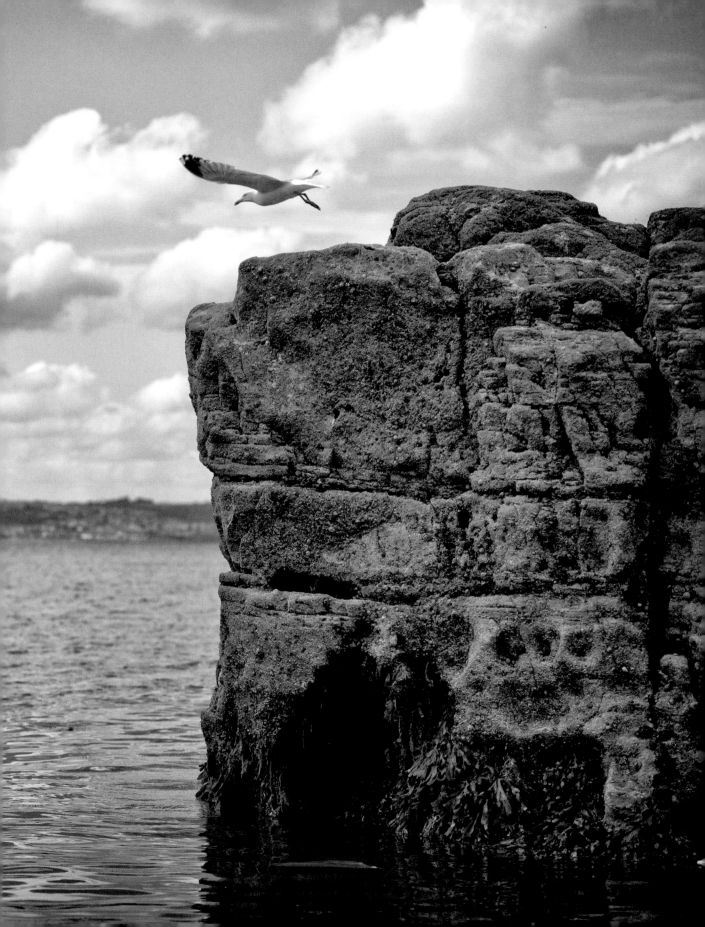

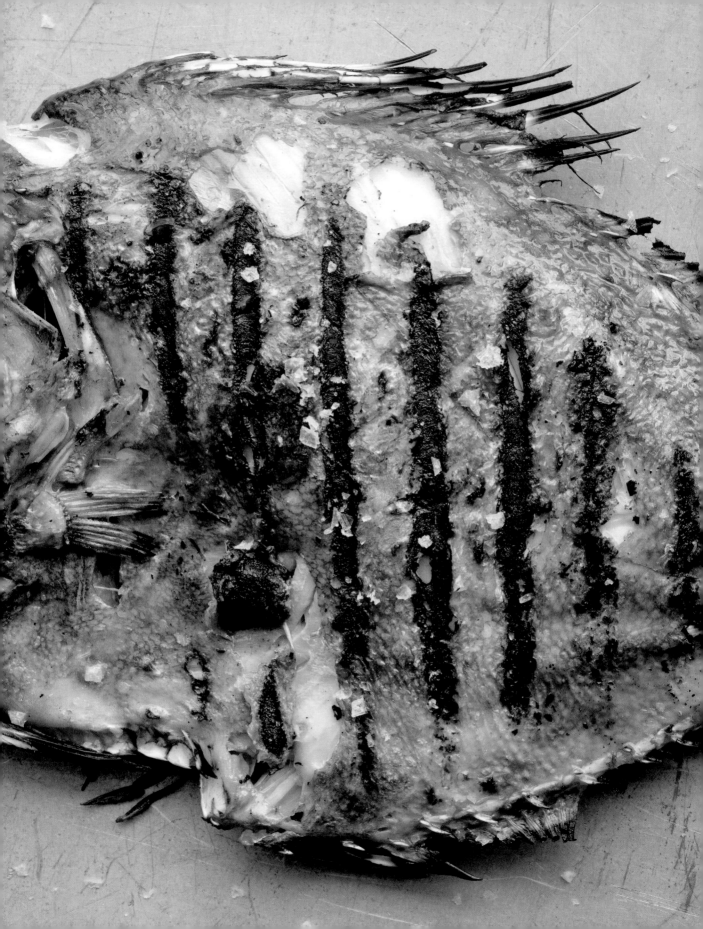

on the grill

the barbecue grill

The best way of grilling fish is over a fire; it produces magnificent results and it's easy to do. You can barbecue whole gutted fish and fillets with equal success. But I would advise against cooking white flaky fish such as cod, pollack and whiting directly on the barbecue grill (instead, these fish can be cooked in a double-lined foil and parchment parcel on the heat with a splash of wine, some butter and herbs). Some fish don't suit being cooked over a fire. Turbot, for instance, suits nothing better than roasting in a conventional oven. Ray, plaice, whiting and any other soft- or large-flaked fish, are best roasted, grilled or cooked in a bag.

tips for successful barbecuing

- Use good-quality charcoal; it will burn for longer and give a better flavour.
- Make sure the barbecue is hot before cooking; allow all flames to die down until you are left with white ash on the coals.
- Brush the grill with a little oil.
- Dry the fish well before putting it on the grill.
- Using the breadcrumb and herb mixture (see page 209) to give the fish a light coating and interesting flavour.

- If you are using a marinade, brush it on the fish as it grills.

- If you are barbecuing a whole fish, tuck herbs such as rosemary, bay or thyme into the belly, and make slashes in the flesh to the bone – this will help reduce the cooking time.

- Try placing an upturned casserole dish over the fish and stoking the fire with herbs such as rosemary and thyme to achieve a lovely smoky, herby flavour.

- If you are barbecuing an oily fish such as mackerel, rub a dry spice mixture onto the fish.

my favourite seafood for barbecuing

Dover sole	Bream	Squid
John Dory	Gurnard	Lobster
Red mullet	Monkfish	Razor clams
Grey mullet	Sardines	Scallops
Sea bass	Mackerel	Prawns
		Langoustines

the flat grill and grill plate

In Spain, the standard method of cooking is on the flat grill or 'plancha'. You can buy flat plates as well as ridged ones for your home hob. (I've also used a big heavy-based frying pan and got it super-hot and had reasonable results.) There is a subtle difference between these cooking methods and the flavours you'll get from them are quite distinct. When you use a ridged grill pan you are touching the fish with fine ridges of very hot metal, which has the effect of 'charring' and giving it that lightly burnt barbecued flavour. On a flat grill the fish builds a crust that has a sweet flavour and golden look; this is an excellent way of cooking shellfish, squid and cuttlefish. When cooking on a flat grill there should be no sign of charring or the flavour will be spoiled. Virtually all seafood works well cooked on a flat grill, but if you are using a ridged grill avoid soft, white flaky fish, whose qualities are best exploited when roasted in an oven.

under the grill

When cooking under the grill, for the best results you need a hot grill; I preheat mine for 10 minutes. Whole oily fish such as mackerel and sardines work particularly well cooked under the grill, as do smaller flatfish such as lemon sole, megrim, Dover sole and dabs. I prefer to skin flatfish before grilling them, but the skin can have good eating qualities when nicely blistered under the grill. If you are going to eat your fish with the skin on, get the fishmonger to remove the scales – although they are not as obvious on flat fish as on round fish, there are scales.

I use a small flat tray, which can be easily pushed under, and removed from, the grill; it also saves you from having to clean the grill tray. Oil it well and place your fish directly on it. Season the fish well and smother it in soft salted butter. The butter ensures a lovely golden crust, but a good smearing of olive oil works well too. Place under the grill for the required cooking time – a Dover sole will take 8–10 minutes, and you can use this as a guide for other flatfish, but it really depends on how hot your grill is. You can add a few herbs such as rosemary or tarragon towards the end of cooking time, or even a smear of garlic butter or anchovy butter over the grilled fish.

John Dory with samphire sauce

SERVES 2

The sauce is based on a recipe by Sarah Raven, a wonderful cook. It's especially good with fish cooked over a fire. I paired it with gutted, skinned and trimmed John Dory (or use tilapia). Preheat the grill (broiler) or barbecue to hot. Brush your fish with olive oil, sprinkle on the herb mix on page 209 and season with sea salt and freshly ground black pepper. Barbecue or grill for 4–6 minutes on each side, skinned side down first, until cooked. To make the sauce, roughly chop a handful of raw marsh samphire, then blitz it in a blender to a purée with 2 tbsp olive oil. Mix in 200 g/7 oz crème fraîche (sour cream) and the juice and zest of 1 unwaxed lemon. Serve the grilled fish with the sauce and lemon wedges.

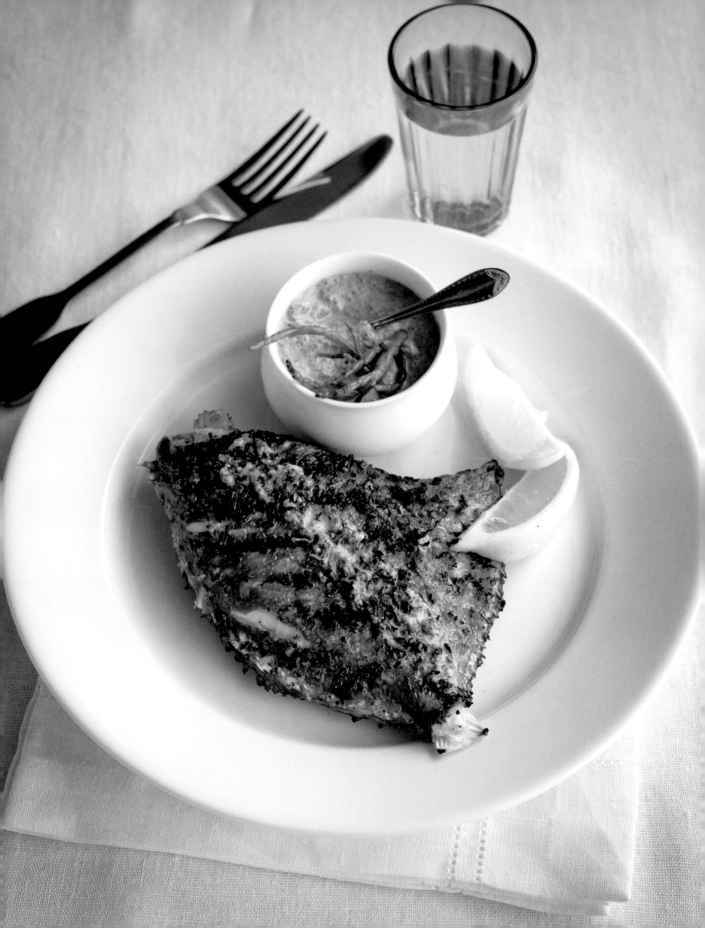

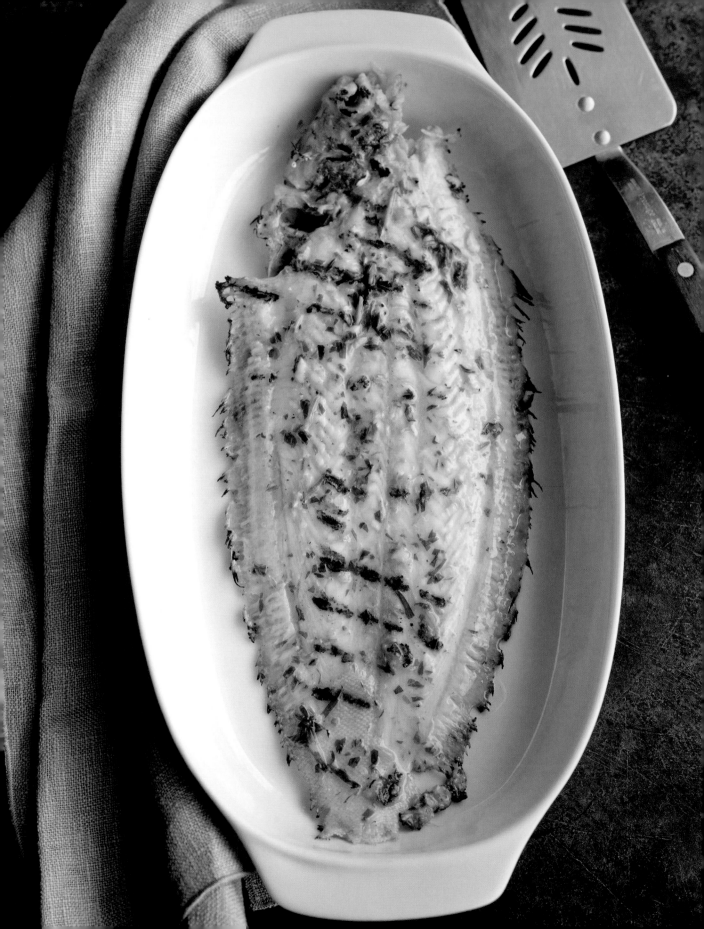

grilled sole with tarragon butter

SERVES 1

Preheat the grill (broiler) to hot. Brush **1 gutted, skinned and trimmed lemon sole, megrim or Dover sole** with **olive oil** and sprinkle with **sea salt** and **black pepper**. Grill (broil) for 8–10 minutes. Blanch **a handful of tarragon leaves**, dry them, then place in a food processor with **100 g/ 3½ oz/scant ½ cup soft butter** and **1 salted anchovy fillet** and blitz until smooth. Dot the tarragon butter over the hot sole. Keep leftover butter in the fridge, wrapped in greaseproof (wax) paper, for brushing over any grilled fish.

AT THE FISHMONGER
Ask your fishmonger to skin, gut and trim 1 sole.

Sorrel has a wonderful affinity with fish. You are most likely to find it between April and early September. If it is not available, use spinach and add a very good squeeze of lemon; it's not quite the same but eats very well.

bream with sorrel and cumin

SERVES 2

400 g/14 oz fresh sorrel leaves (or spinach, but add a good squeeze of lemon), washed well

25 g/1 oz/2 tbsp butter

sea salt and freshly ground black pepper

2 tbsp crème fraîche (sour cream)

pinch of freshly ground cumin

1 sea bream (or red snapper), about 650 g/1 lb 7oz, scaled, filleted and pinboned

flavoured salt (optional)

olive oil

Preheat the grill (broiler) to hot. Very finely slice the sorrel by placing 4–5 leaves on top of each other, rolling them up like a cigar and slicing. Melt the butter in a saucepan over a low heat, add the sorrel and cook until the leaves are wilting. Season and stir in the crème fraîche and cumin.

Season the fish with salt and pepper or a flavoured salt (fennel is my favourite for this dish), then brush with olive oil. Place the fish, skin side up, under the grill for 5–6 minutes until the skin is crisp and the flesh moist and white – bream fillets are thin and there will be no need to turn them. Serve each fillet with a spoonful of sorrel.

AT THE FISHMONGER
Ask your fishmonger to scale, fillet and pinbone
1 x 650 g/1 lb 7 oz sea bream.

grilled gurnard with garlic and wine vinegar

SERVES 2

I love slightly oily fish such as gurnard with piquant flavours from ingredients such as capers and lemon. Here the fish is grilled (broiled) and served with a simple sauce. Preheat your grill to hot. Brush 2 x 200 g/7 oz gurnard fillets with olive oil and sprinkle with a little sea salt. Grill (broil) them for 6–8 minutes, until cooked. Place a frying pan over a medium-high heat, add 8 tbsp olive oil and, when hot, add 2 finely sliced garlic cloves and cook for 1–2 minutes, until turning golden. Add 3 tbsp good white wine vinegar or lemon or lime juice, allow the vinegar to boil off, then add 1 tbsp finely chopped curly parsley and spoon over the fish.

This makes a nice shared starter for two – or simply double the ingredients for four. Around August time, just after the small squid have come inshore, the small red mullet follow and they are relatively inexpensive for about six weeks. This also works well with a handful of crab meat added to the salad.

grilled red mullet with cucumber and coriander

SERVES 2 TO START

2 small red mullet (or red snapper), scaled, filleted and pinboned

100 ml/3½ fl oz/½ cup olive oil, plus a little extra for brushing the fish

sea salt and freshly ground black pepper

pinch of freshly ground cumin

pinch of caster (superfine) sugar

juice of 1 lime or lemon

¼ cucumber, peeled, deseeded, quartered and thinly sliced

4 radishes, thinly sliced

small handful of fresh coriander (cilantro), roughly chopped

6 spring onions (scallions), cut into fine julienne

Preheat the grill (broiler) to hot. Brush the mullet fillets with olive oil and season with salt and pepper. Grill (broil), skin side up, until blistered and golden and cooked through – this will take 3–4 minutes.

To make the dressing, mix the olive oil and cumin with the sugar and lime or lemon juice, taste to check that the acidity is balanced. Place the remaining ingredients, including the fish, into a bowl and season well, then pour the dressing over and, using your hands, make sure everything is well dressed and the fish just broken lightly into the salad. Serve on a plate to share.

AT THE FISHMONGER
Ask your fishmonger to scale, fillet and pinbone 2 small red mullet.

grilled red mullet with Adriatic dressing

SERVES 1

Preheat the grill (broiler) to hot. Brush a **scaled and gutted red mullet** (or **red snapper**) with **sea salt** and **olive oil**. Make a cut or two in one side and insert a **bay leaf** into each cut. Grill for 4–5 minutes on each side, depending on the size of the fish. Make the dressing by crumbling **100 g/ 3½ oz feta cheese** into **3–4 tbsp crème fraîche** (sour cream), add lots of finely **chopped fresh dill,** **1 tbsp roughly chopped black olives** and plenty of **black pepper.** Serve alongside the fish with a simple **tomato and red onion salad** dressed with **basil, olive oil** and plenty of **sea salt.**

AT THE FISHMONGER
Ask your fishmonger to scale and gut a red mullet.

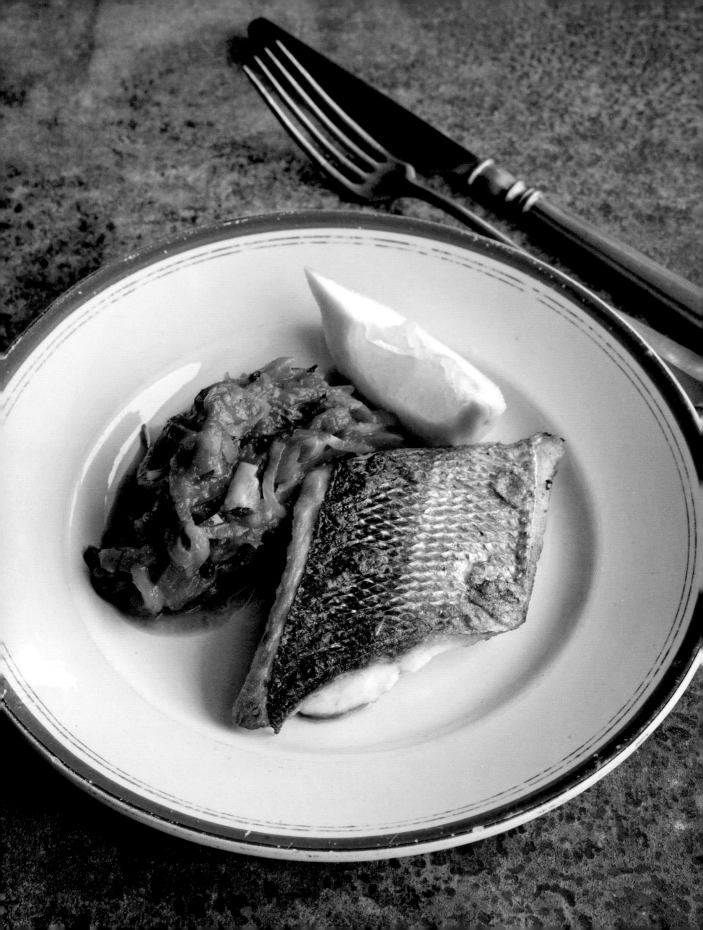

My best pal and chef 'Mat the clam' at The Seahorse restaurant makes a fine peperonata. It's great with any fish and works especially well with bass, tuna and hake.

sea bass with peperonata and basil

SERVES 4

2 sea bass, each about
450 g/1 lb, scaled, filleted and
pinboned
sea salt and freshly ground black
pepper
olive oil
2 garlic cloves, finely chopped
2 red onions, finely sliced
sprig of thyme, leaves picked
1 tbsp tomato purée
3 tomatoes, peeled, deseeded and
roughly chopped
2 red (bell) peppers, deseeded and
finely sliced
pinch of saffron strands
good pinch of freshly ground cumin
1 tbsp red wine or red wine vinegar
a few fresh basil leaves, roughly torn
juice of 1 lemon, plus lemon wedges
to serve

First make a few slashes diagonally in the skin of the sea bass about 2.5 cm/1 in apart, season with a sprinkling of salt and set aside.

To make the peperonata, heat 5–6 tbsp olive oil in a pan, add the garlic, onions and thyme and cook gently over a low heat for 10–15 minutes without colouring. Add the tomato purée and cook for 1–2 minutes, then add the tomatoes and red peppers and cook gently for 25 minutes, until softened and the whole mixture is really stewed down. Add the saffron and cumin and continue to cook for 5 minutes, then add the red wine or red wine vinegar to balance the sweetness. Preheat the grill (broiler) to hot.

To cook the fish, brush with olive oil, then grill (broil), skin side facing the heat, without turning (unless the fillets are thick) for 6–7 minutes.

Warm the peperonata and stir in a few basil leaves and a little squeeze of lemon. Season and serve alongside the fish, with a lemon wedge.

AT THE FISHMONGER
Ask your fishmonger to scale, fillet and pinbone 2 x 450 g/1 lb sea bass.

I picked up this recipe on the Adriatic coast of the region of Emilia-Romagna in Italy. It's a typical way of preparing fish for grilling (broiling) in Italy and we often use it at my restaurant The Seahorse. It's especially good if you are cooking over coals, but it also works well on a grill plate or under a conventional grill.

monkfish as grilled in Romagna

SERVES 4 TO START

100 ml/3½ fl oz/½ cup dry white wine

4 tbsp olive oil

1 monkfish tail, about 650 g/1 lb 7 oz, skin and membrane removed

sea salt and freshly ground black pepper

1 tbsp dried oregano

1 tbsp fennel seeds

½ tbsp dried thyme

4 bay leaves, roughly ground

small handful of fine fresh breadcrumbs

1 dried bird's-eye chilli (chile), crushed

Mix the wine with the olive oil in a dish. Sprinkle the fish with salt and pepper, then add to the dish, turn to coat and leave to marinate for 15 minutes.

Meanwhile, mix the oregano, fennel, thyme, bay, breadcrumbs and chilli together.

Preheat the grill (broiler) to hot. Sprinkle the fish lightly with the herb and breadcrumb mixture and grill (broil) for 10–15 minutes, turning halfway through and allowing each side to blacken.

AT THE FISHMONGER
Ask your fishmonger to remove the skin and membrane from
1 x 650 g/1 lb 7 oz monkfish tail.

grilled mackerel with lemon, ginger and basil

SERVES 2

Preheat the grill (broiler) or grill pan to hot. Make a few slashes diagonally down one side of each of 2 gutted and deheaded mackerel, then rub with sea salt and olive oil. Grill (broil) for 4–5 minutes on each side.

Roughly chop an unwaxed lemon and put it in a food processor with 2 tbsp caster (superfine) sugar, a good grind of black pepper, 1 cm/½ in peeled root ginger and 6–7 basil leaves. Blitz for 1 minute until smooth, then serve with the grilled mackerel. Wonderful, zingy and perfect for cutting through the delicious oils in the fish.

AT THE FISHMONGER
Ask your fishmonger to gut and dehead 2 mackerel.

grilled mackerel with spiced salt

SERVES 2

Fresh out of the water, there couldn't be a finer fish than mackerel, especially when thrown onto a grill. Preheat the grill (broiler) to hot. Make a few cuts in each side of **2 gutted and deheaded mackerel**, going down to the bone. Mix together **2 tbsp rock salt, 1 tbsp ground star anise** and **½ tbsp freshly ground Sichuan peppercorns**. Rub into the fish, brush with **olive oil** and grill (broil) for 3–4 minutes on each side, until blackened and crisp. Finish with a **squeeze of lime** and enjoy the numbing sensation from the peppercorns.

AT THE FISHMONGER
Ask your fishmonger to gut and dehead 2 mackerel.

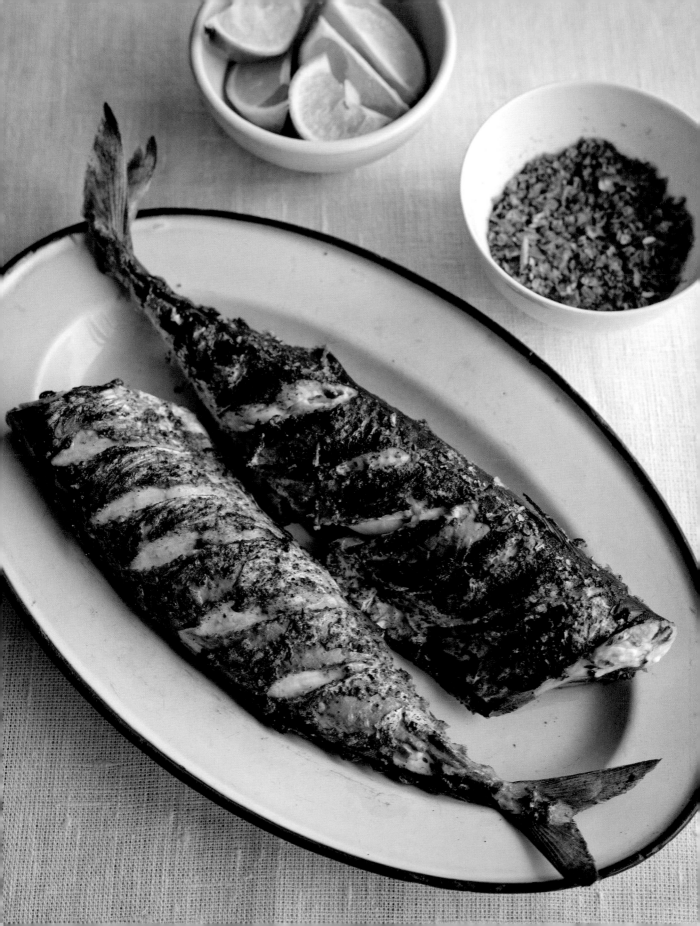

grilled sardines with fennel seeds and black pepper

SERVES 1

Fennel seeds and black pepper are a delightful combination. Preheat the grill (broiler) to hot. Grind 1 tbsp fennel seeds and 1 tbsp black pepper with a little sea salt. Rub into 3–4 gutted sardines, and brush with olive oil. Grill (broil) them for 2–3 minutes on each side, until blistering and crisp with their wonderful oils oozing everywhere. A big plate of these with a few wedges of lemon is just fine as it is.

AT THE FISHMONGER
Ask your fishmonger to gut 3–4 sardines.

If you can't get octopus, make the sauce and use it on mackerel, tuna or even monkfish. This is best cooked over coals, but you can grill (broil) it if you prefer.

grilled octopus with barbecue sauce

SERVES 4 TO START

1 frozen octopus, about 1 kg/2 lb 4 oz

1 bay leaf

1 tbsp olive oil

For the barbecue sauce

100 ml/3½ fl oz/½ cup tomato ketchup

1 tsp ground fennel seeds

2 tbsp caster (superfine) sugar

1½ tbsp Dijon mustard

1 tbsp white wine vinegar

Tabasco to taste

good grind of black pepper and sea salt, to taste

1 tbsp ras el hanout

2 tsp light soy sauce

1 garlic clove, finely chopped

1 tbsp finely chopped fresh flat-leaf parsley

100 ml/3½ fl oz/½ cup runny honey

juice and zest of 1 unwaxed lemon

pinch of hot chilli (chile) powder

First thaw the octopus, covered, overnight in the fridge. Cook it in the morning of the day you need it. Place it in a large pan with the bay leaf and olive oil. Place over a low heat, cover and simmer for about 1 hour – the octopus will release its juices and cook in them. To test if it is cooked, insert a knife into a thick part of a tentacle – it should feel like cooked potato and the knife should easily go in and out. Allow to cool, then place in the fridge to 'set'.

To make the sauce (you can do this in advance), put all the ingredients into a pan and simmer gently over a low heat while stirring. Balance the flavours by adding more sugar or salt to taste, then cook at a gentle simmer until the sauce has the same consistency as HP sauce – about 10 minutes.

Fire up the barbecue (before cooking, ensure the flames have died down and the coals are glowing and covered with white ash) or preheat the grill (broiler) to very hot. Separate the octopus tentacles from the body and rub off any loose purple skin. Cut into large chunks, thread onto metal skewers and brush with the barbecue sauce. Cook, basting all the time, turning from time to time, for about 5 minutes. The sauce will be sweet, salty and form a sticky coating on the octopus.

AT THE FISHMONGER

If you have a good fishmonger, ask him to source the 'double sucker' variety of octopus, he will know what you mean. They come frozen, cleaned and weigh about 1 kg/2 lb 4 oz, just enough for 4 people.

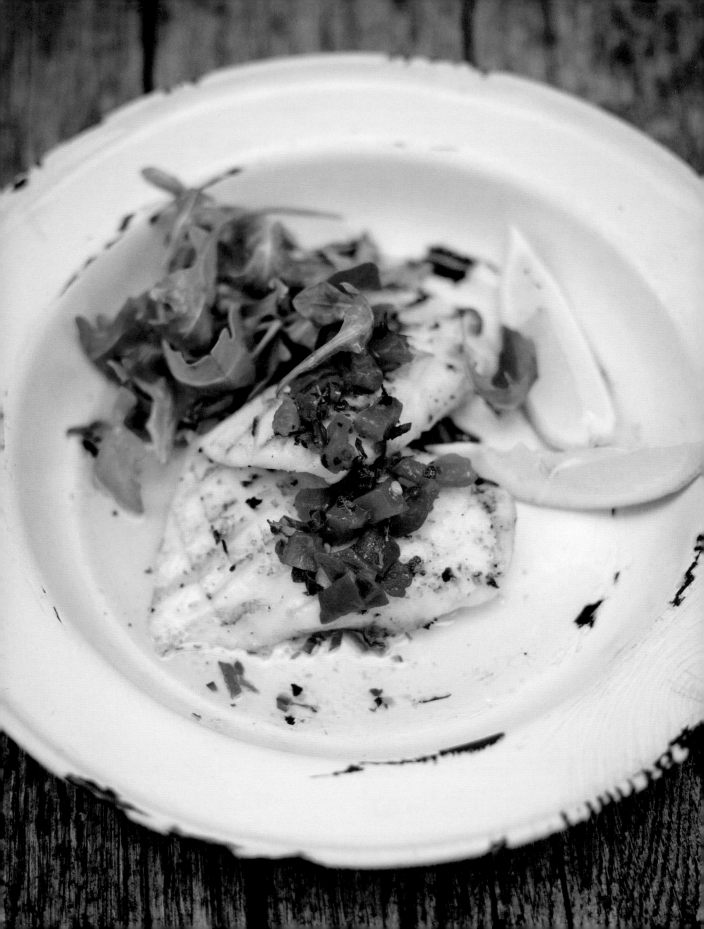

Squid (calamari) is a big favourite of mine. A very versatile seafood, it's equally wonderful simply fried or slow-braised with wine and herbs; in each preparation it takes on different qualities. Grilled squid, especially cooked over a fire, is unique too. The squid is scored from the inside so that not only does it curl and look good, but also the little knobbles of squid catch the heat source or fire and the flavour is magnificent.

grilled squid with oregano and chilli

SERVES 4

4 squid (calamari), each about 150 g/5½ oz, cleaned and skinned

olive oil

sea salt and freshly ground black pepper

2 tsp fennel seeds, finely ground

2 small handfuls of fine fresh breadcrumbs

2 handfuls of rocket (arugula) to serve

juice of ½ lemon, plus lemon wedges to serve

For the dressing

4 mild red chillies (chiles), deseeded and finely diced

1 small dried bird's-eye chilli (chile)

1 red (bell) pepper, roasted, peeled, deseeded and finely chopped

2 tomatoes, skinned, deseeded and finely chopped

1 tbsp finely chopped fresh oregano

1 tbsp finely chopped fresh curly parsley

pinch of dried oregano

1 tbsp good-quality white wine vinegar with some sweetness

100 ml/3½ fl oz/½ cup olive oil

Preheat the grill to hot – whether it's an overhead grill (broiler), grill plate or barbecue (if a barbecue, ensure the flames have died down and the coals are glowing and covered with white ash before cooking).

Slice the squid from top to bottom, then open it out and make diagonal cuts across it first one way and then the other, making sure the depth of the cut is just halfway through the thickness of the squid. Brush with olive oil and season with salt and pepper, then sprinkle with the fennel seeds and breadcrumbs. Place under the grill, cut side facing the heat – the squid will curl on itself, and cook until golden and evenly charred on the knobbly bits – for 6–8 minutes.

To make the dressing, mix together all the ingredients (you can sweeten your vinegar if necessary with a little caster/superfine sugar), taste to balance the flavours and season – sweet, hot, and aromatic from the oregano is what you are looking for.

To serve, place the squid on a plate and spoon the dressing liberally over it. Dress the rocket with a little olive oil and lemon juice, season and serve with the squid and lemon wedges.

AT THE FISHMONGER
Ask your fishmonger to clean and skin 4 squid.

I'm no expert on Asian food, but I love it. I relish trips to Australia to eat with some of the chefs there who have the most amazing understanding of Asian flavours. This very simple dish was shown to me by my pal John Susman. He's my fish guru in the southern hemisphere and we have travelled a lot together in search of the finest seafood experiences. I think we both agree that cuttlefish would be amongst them. This sauce is also very good with prawns (shrimp). I recommend waiting for good weather and cooking this over a fire.

cuttlefish with John Susman's nam jim sauce

SERVES 4

small handful of fresh coriander (cilantro) with stalks

3 garlic cloves

2 red chillies (chiles), deseeded and finely chopped

sea salt

2 shallots, finely chopped (small Thai red ones are best)

2 tbsp fish sauce

juice of 1 lime

2 tbsp grated palm sugar

3 medium cuttlefish, cleaned and prepared

olive oil

1. Preheat the grill to hot, or fire up the barbecue (if barbecuing, ensure the flames have died down and the coals are glowing and covered with white ash before cooking).

AT THE FISHMONGER
Ask your fishmonger to clean and prepare 3 cuttlefish.

2. Make the nam jim. Crush the coriander, garlic, chillies and salt to taste to a paste in a pestle and mortar.

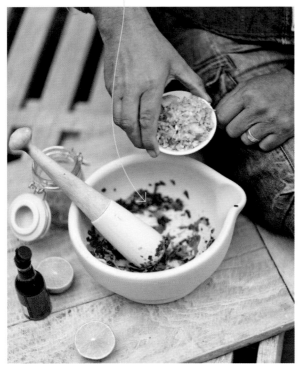

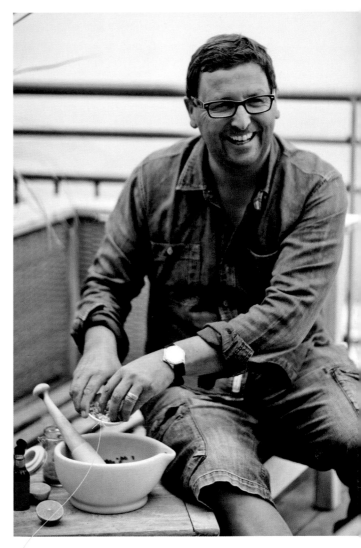

3. Throw in the shallots and crush.

4. Add the fish sauce, lime juice and sugar to taste and balance the flavours by adding more of any of these ingredients – you want salty, sweet and hot.

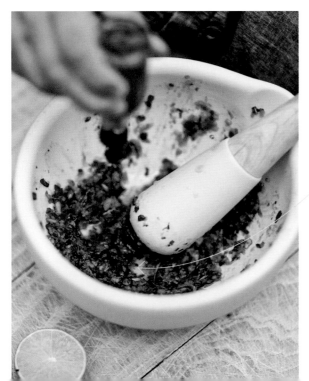

5. Slice the cuttlefish from top to bottom and lay it flat. Using the tip of a sharp knife, make diagonal cuts about 1 cm/½ in apart, first one way and then the other, on the inside of the cuttlefish, making sure the depth of the cut is just halfway through the thickness.

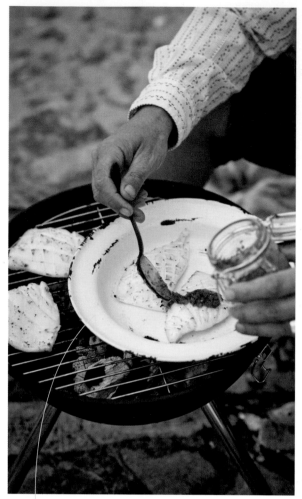

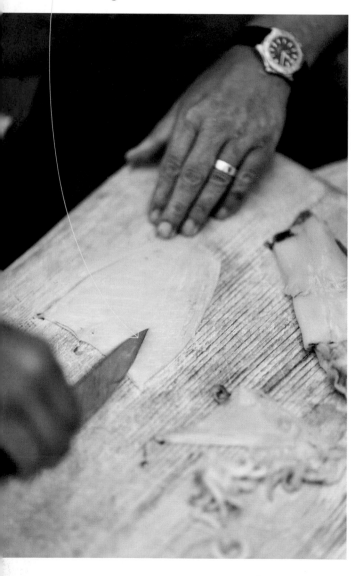

6. Brush with olive oil and season with salt, then grill or cook over coals, with the cut side nearest the heat, until charred and golden – about 8 minutes. Spoon the dressing liberally over the fish and serve.

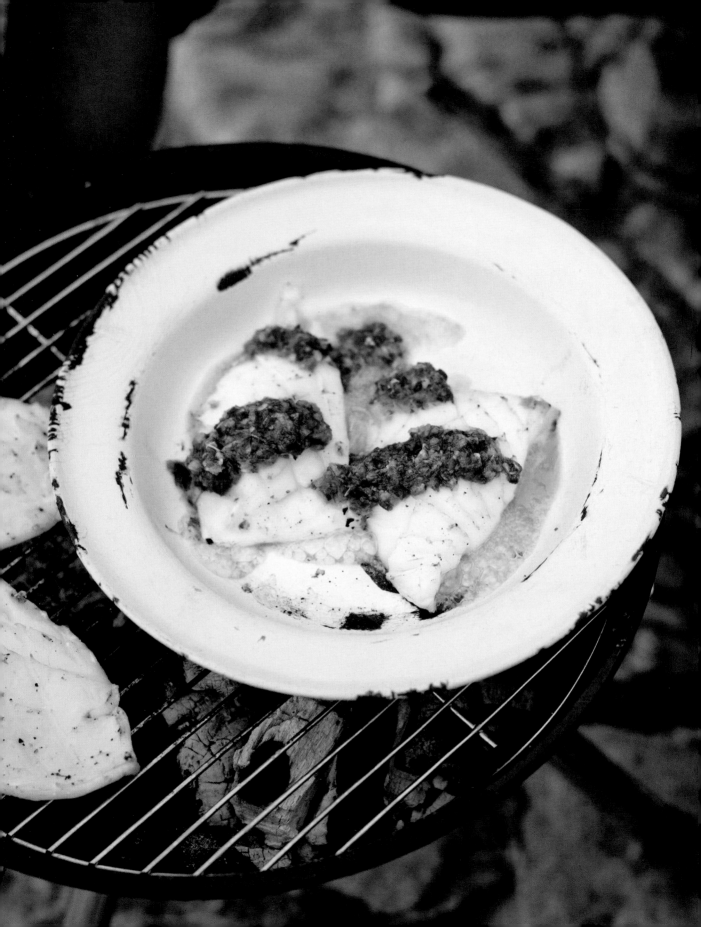

It doesn't get much simpler than this, but the right choice of seafood can ensure that it will be heavenly. If you can, cook the seafood over a fire, but a grill plate will also give you great results. I dress the fish with a little olive oil seasoned with salt and mixed with parsley, but you could try the dressing from the squid recipe on page 37, the salsa Milanese on page 57, or the nam jim sauce on page 38 – they all make wonderful sauces for grilled fish (or, for a special occasion, you might like to try all three). My favourite selection of fish is below, but use the best of what you can buy at the fish counter.

mixed grill of seafood

SERVES 2

1 live lobster, about 600 g/1 lb 5 oz

1 medium squid (calamari), cleaned and prepared

1 John Dory (or tilapia), about 350 g/12 oz, scaled, gutted, fins and tail trimmed and deheaded

a couple of slices of monkfish, cut across the tail through the bone, leaving the bone in

a few raw prawns with the shell on

olive oil

sea salt and freshly ground black pepper

1–2 tbsp herb mixture for grilling (see page 209)

handful of flat-leaf parsley, finely chopped to garnish

lemon wedges and your choice of dressing (see introduction) to serve

Place the lobster on a chopping board. Insert a large, sharp, heavy knife into the cross on the back of the head and cut down towards the tail, cutting it in half. Remove the stomach and the black intestinal tract (if there is one) that may run through the middle of the tail and discard. Slice the squid from top to bottom, then open it out and make diagonal cuts across it, first one way and then the other, making sure the depth of the cut is halfway through the thickness.

Preheat the barbecue, or the grill (broiler), to hot. (If barbecuing, ensure the flames have died down and the coals are glowing and covered with white ash before cooking.) Brush all the prepared fish and shellfish with olive oil, season and sprinkle with the grill mixture. Gently grill the squid, cut side down over the hot coals, or cut side up under the grill (the squid will curl up on itself) until golden and evenly charred on the knobbly bits – about 5 minutes. Gently grill the lobster, flesh side down over the hot coals, or flesh side up under the grill, for 5 minutes, then turn it over and cook for a further 4–5 minutes – it should be nicely scorched and grilled. Meawhile, put the monkfish and John Dory on or under the grill and cook until nicely charred – about 4 minutes on each side. Grill the prawns for 4–5 minutes until pink.

Place all the fish on a big platter, sprinkle with parsley and sea salt and serve with a few lemon wedges and your choice of dressing. One of my favourite meals of all time.

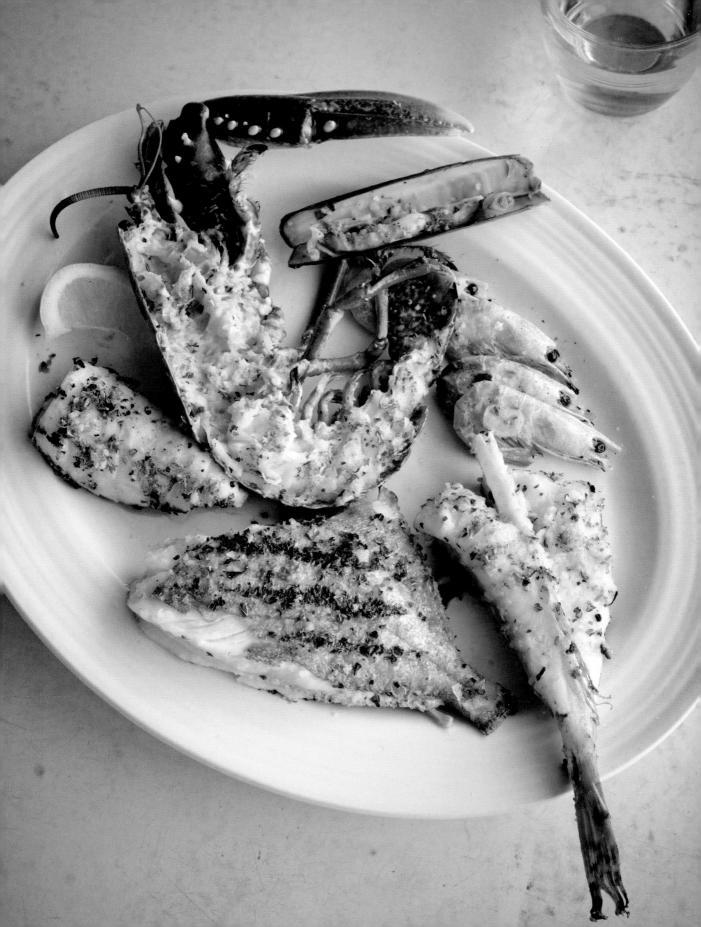

Lobster is great grilled over coals; it also works well cooked under a grill (broiler) or on a grill plate.

grilled lobster with chilli and rosemary

SERVES 2

I live lobster, about 750 g/1 lb 10 oz
1 tbsp roughly chopped fresh rosemary
1 tbsp roughly chopped fresh flat-leaf parsley
1 red chilli (chile), deseeded and roughly chopped
2 garlic cloves
1 dried red bird's-eye chilli (chile)
sea salt and freshly ground black pepper to taste
150 g/5½ oz/¾ cup butter, softened
juice of 1 lemon

1. Preheat the grill or barbecue to hot. Place the lobster on a chopping board. Insert a large, sharp, heavy knife into the cross on the back of the head and cut down towards the tail, cutting it in half. Remove the stomach and the black intestinal tract (if there is one) that may run through the middle of the tail and discard. Place all the remaining ingredients (including salt and pepper to taste) except the butter and lemon juice in a food processor and blitz until you have a smooth paste, then add the butter and lemon juice and blitz for 1 minute.

2. Season the lobster, then place under the grill, flesh side up, or if using a grill plate or barbecue flesh side down, and cook for 4–5 minutes.

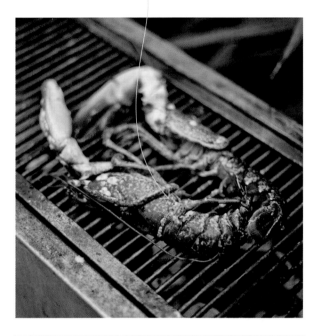

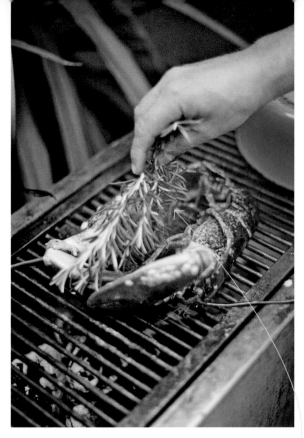

3. Brush the flesh with the butter mixture. If cooking on a barbecue, stoke the fire with a rosemary sprig.

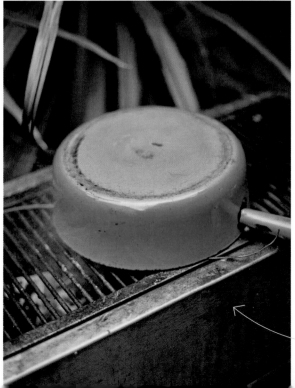

4. If cooking on a barbecue, place an upturned heavy casserole over the top of the lobster to give it a lovely smoky, herby flavour.

5. Keep basting the lobster until it is cooked through, which should take no longer than a further 5-6 minutes.

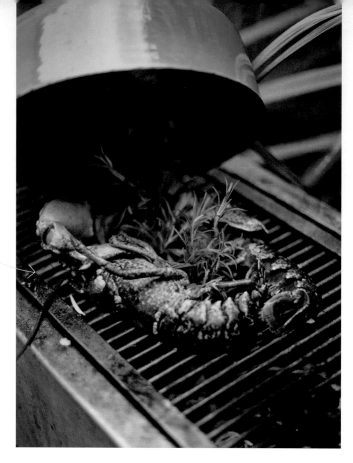

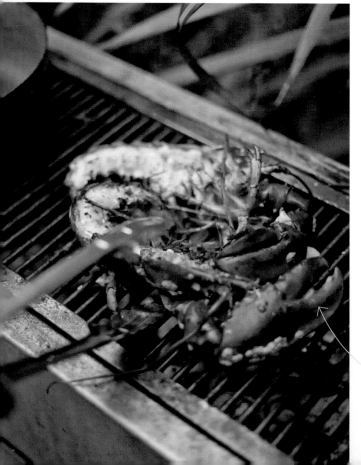

6. Serve with a simple salad of leaves – rocket is my favourite – dressed with lemon juice and olive oil.

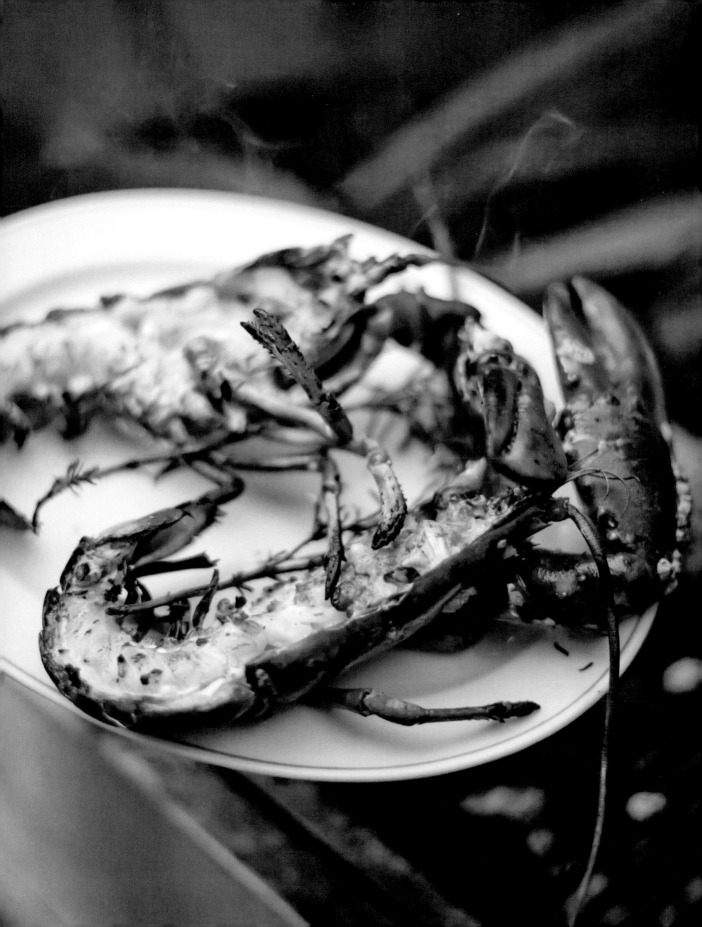

Spider crab may be hard to find but it is worth seeking out. Try to buy the meat only, as it's time-consuming to pick from the shell. The cooked meat is so good it's worth eating it dressed simply with olive oil and lemon juice and a few lettuce leaves, but this dish is superb too. It can be made equally successfully with meat from the more common brown crab. I like to serve this in the shell, as the final grilling heats the shell and you get some wonderful aromas from it. If you have no shells, small gratin dishes or scallop shells work fine.

grilled spider crab as cooked in Spain

SERVES 2

olive oil

2 tbsp finely chopped leeks

8 cherry tomatoes, quartered

½ garlic clove, crushed to a paste

2 tbsp finely chopped celery

1 tbsp dry sherry

1 tbsp brandy

60 g/2¼ oz cooked brown spider crab meat

a few fresh tarragon leaves, chopped

50 ml/2 fl oz/4 tbsp double (heavy) cream

sea salt and freshly ground black pepper

150 g/5½ oz cooked white spider crab meat

handful of fine fresh breadcrumbs

small knob of butter

1 tsp finely chopped fresh curly parsley

lemon wedges to serve

Preheat the grill (broiler) to hot. Heat 1 tbsp olive oil in a pan, add the leeks, tomatoes, garlic and celery and cook over a low heat until softened, about 4 minutes. Increase the heat, add the sherry and boil off, then add the brandy and boil off again. Stir in the brown crab meat and tarragon, then add the cream, taste and season and take off the heat. Stir in the white crab meat.

Pour into the shells or dishes, sprinkle the top with breadcrumbs add a small knob of butter and brown under the grill. Sprinkle with the parsley and serve with lemon wedges.

AT THE FISHMONGER
Ask your fishmonger for the crab meat only, as it's time-consuming to pick from the shell.

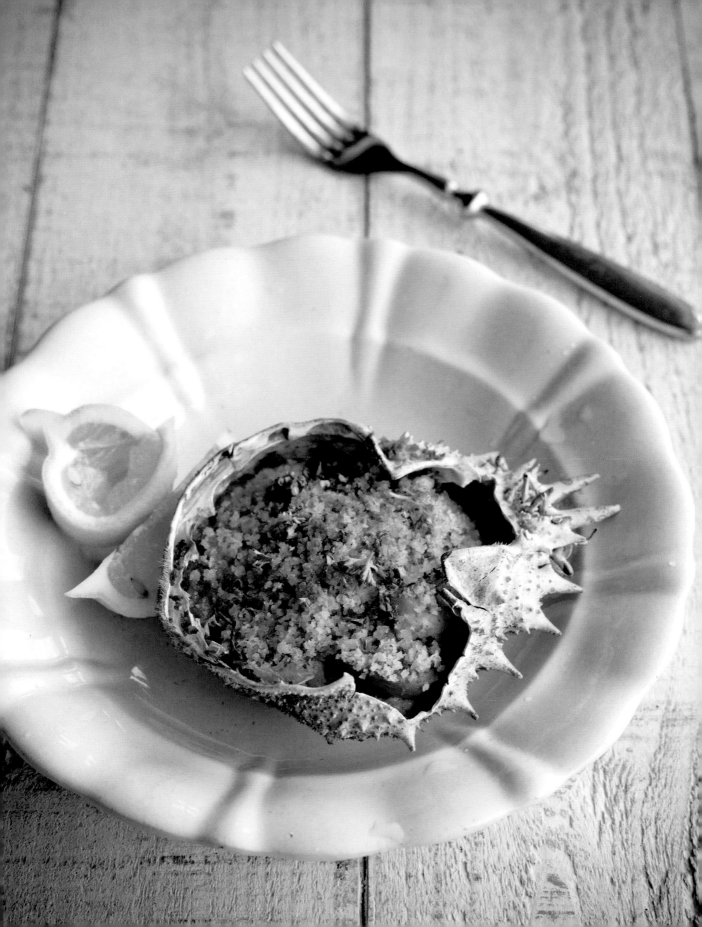

sauces and dressings for grilled seafood

Once you've mastered grilling fish you will find it's very easy and the difference between the seafood dishes you eat will be the individual qualities of the fish itself and, of course, what you dress it with. A few herbs tucked into the belly of a fish will always make a difference too. Here are some of my favourite sauces and dressings; they work every time with a simple piece of grilled fish and will transform it into something extraordinary.

At my restaurant we ensure we have really good olive oils and vinegars to hand – when cooking so simply it really is all about the ingredients. Some vinegars are sweet, some are thicker and all have different uses and very different flavours. I advise buying good vinegar and oil for use at home.

garlic, lemon and parsley dressing

SERVES 2

Season 6 tbsp good olive oil with sea salt and freshly ground black pepper. Stir in 1 crushed garlic clove and 1 tbsp finely chopped fresh flat-leaf parsley. Mix in lemon juice to taste.

chilli, parsley and roast pepper sauce

SERVES 2

Roast **1–2 red (bell) peppers,** depending on size, in the oven or in a flame until blackened, then put them in a plastic tub with the lid on for 15 minutes to allow them to finish cooking and soften. Remove the skin and seeds, strain the juices and reserve. Cut the pepper flesh into fine dice and mix with the reserved juices, **8 tbsp good olive oil, sea salt and freshly ground black pepper** and **1 finely chopped red chilli (chile).** Add **3 tbsp sweet vinegar** and **3 tbsp finely chopped fresh flat-leaf parsley.**

anchovy sauce

SERVES 2

Place 6 salted anchovy fillets, 1 tsp capers,
1 garlic clove, the juice and zest of 1 unwaxed
lemon, 1 tbsp finely chopped fresh flat-leaf
parsley, freshly ground black pepper and 1 small
chopped shallot in a food processor and blitz
until smooth. Add 5 tbsp olive oil with the
motor running to make an emulsion.

Niçoise dressing

Finely chop 6–8 cherry tomatoes, 6 black olives, 1 small artichoke heart and 1 tbsp torn fresh basil, mix together in a bowl, then dress with 4 tbsp olive oil. Season and stir in a squeeze of lemon juice.

oregano and chilli dressing

SERVES 2

Finely chop 1 tbsp fresh oregano and 2 small dried chillies (chiles). Mix into 6 tbsp good olive oil and season with sea salt and plenty of freshly ground black pepper. Add 2 tbsp good red wine vinegar and a pinch of dried oregano.

chilli, mint and coriander yogurt sauce

SERVES 1

Put ½ roughly chopped red onion into a food processor with a handful of fresh coriander (cilantro) leaves, a handful of fresh mint leaves and 1 deseeded and finely chopped green chilli (chile). Add 200 ml/7 fl oz/scant 1 cup natural yogurt and blitz for 1–2 minutes, until you have a smooth sauce. Finish with a squeeze of lime juice. Great with grilled mackerel.

salsa Milanese

SERVES 2

Chop 1 tbsp capers, 3–4 salted anchovy fillets,
1 garlic clove and 1 tbsp fresh basil together, mix
with a small handful of fresh white breadcrumbs.
Moisten with 3 tbsp sweet white wine vinegar and
then add 4 tbsp olive oil and season with sea salt
and freshly ground black pepper. Leave to stand
for a few minutes to allow the crumbs to soak it
all up – it should be spoonable.

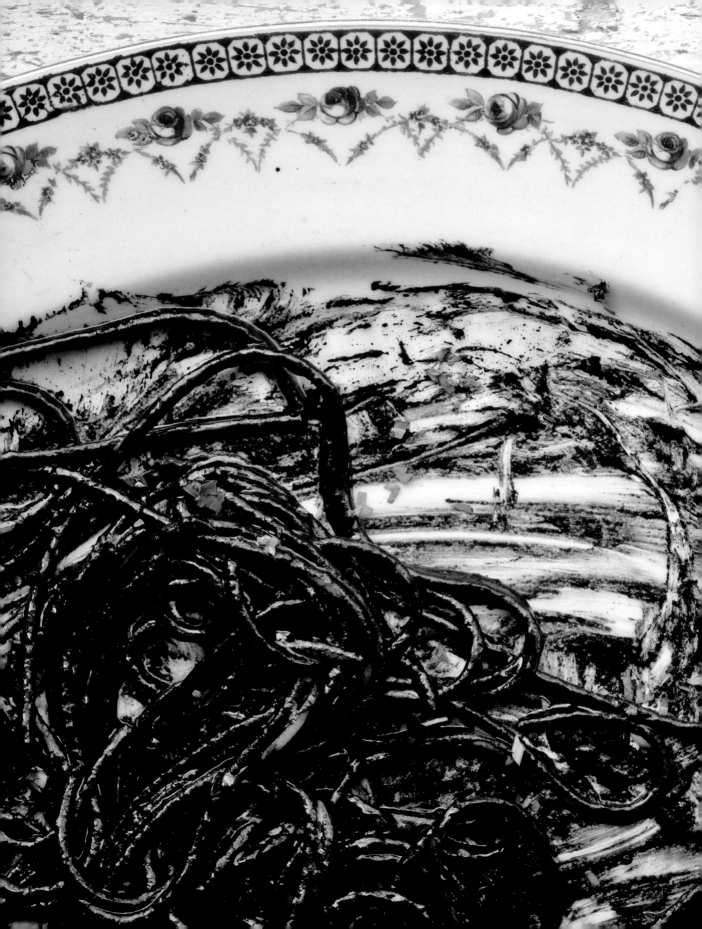

in the pan

frying fish

This is the method most people use when cooking fish. I use a good, heavy-based non-stick pan. I get it nice and hot, then add a tablespoon of two of vegetable or olive oil (extra virgin olive oil is not necessary). When it's hot, season your fish and lay it in the pan, presentation side down – that is, the side you will eventually serve uppermost. Let it cook for 2–3 minutes and then, using a pair of tongs or a fish slice, turn it over; you should have a nice golden finish to it.

If you're cooking a thick fillet of white fish such as cod or pollack, or a steak of turbot or brill, it will also need time in the oven (see the oven chapter, from page 98). Before you start to cook, preheat the oven to maximum. When the fish has taken on colour in the pan, either pop the whole pan in the oven (if it has an overproof handle) or transfer the fish to a roasting pan and put that in the oven – allow 8–10 minutes to cook a piece of fish, depending on the size of course.

For a more luxurious result when cooking in the pan, use lots of butter. A sole or fillet of gurnard, brill or turbot works exceptionally well when cooked like this. Lightly flour the fish, then give it a few taps to remove any excess flour. Heat a small amount of vegetable oil in the pan and, when hot, add the fish and cook for a few minutes. Check the underside to see if it has coloured, then turn it over and add 85 g/3 oz/6 tbsp soft salted butter. When the butter starts to foam, tip the pan towards you and spoon the foaming butter continuously over the fish for 4–5 minutes. You can, if you like, add a few sage or parsley leaves and a squeeze of lemon. Serve the fish with a tablespoon of the butter.

You will often see this on menus in Venice described as '*Sfogi* (sole) *in Saor*'; although it is commonly made with other fish such as mackerel and langoustines. The trick is to get a sweet and sour flavour from cooking the onions until sweet, then balancing the dish with the sharpness of vinegar. This should be served at room temperature and it makes an ideal plate for a lunch served family-style or as an antipasti. You can use any type of sole, including megrim, sand sole, dab, lemon sole, or the expensive but delicious Dover sole.

sole fillets as prepared in Venice

SERVES 4

olive oil

2 large onions, finely chopped

1 bay leaf

2 tbsp plain (all-purpose) flour

2 sole, each about 450 g/1 lb, filleted and skinned

50 g/2 oz/¼ cup caster (superfine) sugar

100 ml/3½ fl oz/½ cup good-quality white wine vinegar

1 tbsp pine nuts, lightly toasted

sea salt and freshly ground black pepper

handful of fresh flat-leaf parsley, finely chopped

green salad to serve

Heat 2 tbsp olive oil in a saucepan. Add the onions and bay leaf, cover and sweat over a low heat for about 40 minutes.

Meanwhile, put the flour in a shallow bowl and dip the sole fillets into it to lightly flour them. Heat 5 tbsp olive oil in a frying pan over a low-medium heat. When it's hot, add the fish and fry for 2 minutes on each side, until lightly golden, then set aside on a serving platter.

Remove the lid from the onions, add the sugar and cook until golden, then add the vinegar and cook for a further 4–5 minutes – the taste should balance sweetness from the onions and acidity from the vinegar. Stir in the pine nuts, taste for seasoning, then spoon this mixture over the sole fillets and sprinkle with parsley. Serve at room temperature. Excellent with a simple green salad.

AT THE FISHMONGER
Ask your fishmonger to fillet and skin 2 x 450 g/1 lb sole.

Gurnard is an amazing fish, especially the larger tub gurnard. It is wonderful for roasting and braising and is particularly delightful in this simple stew with leeks and oysters.

gurnard with oysters and leeks

SERVES 2

olive oil for frying

2 gurnard fillets, each about 200 g/7 oz, pinboned

2 leeks, finely sliced

200 ml/7 fl oz/scant 1 cup double (heavy) cream

1 tbsp English mustard

pinch of cayenne

sea salt and freshly ground black pepper

6 oysters, shucked

1 tbsp finely chopped fresh tarragon

Heat a frying pan, add a little olive oil and, when it's hot, add the gurnard, skin side down, and fry until crisp. Cook the leeks gently in a saucepan in their own moisture until soft but not coloured. Add them to the gurnard, then add the cream, mustard and cayenne and season with salt and plenty of freshly ground black pepper. Simmer for 4–5 minutes, then add the oysters and cook gently for a further 3 minutes. Sprinkle with tarragon and serve. You should have a thick creamy sauce to spoon over the fish.

AT THE FISHMONGER
Ask your fishmonger to scale, fillet and pinbone gunard.

Red mullet has a unique flavour – the skin has a hint of saffron and shellfish and the flesh is white and slightly oily. I like to cook it as simply as possible.

red mullet with anchovy and sage

SERVES 2

plain (all-purpose) flour for dusting

2 red mullet (or red snapper), each about 200 g/7 oz, scaled, filleted and pinboned

olive oil

2 tbsp dry white wine

2 salted anchovy fillets, finely chopped

6–7 fresh sage leaves

handful of coarse fresh breadcrumbs

1 tbsp finely chopped fresh flat-leaf parsley

freshly ground black pepper

squeeze of lemon juice

Lightly flour the mullet fillets and shallow-fry, skin side down, in a little olive oil over a medium-high heat until crisp and golden – 3–4 minutes – then turn them and cook for a few more minutes until they are cooked through. Transfer the fish to warm plates.

Add the wine to the pan and stir to pick up all the crispy bits; boil for a second or two, then add a few tablespoons of olive oil and heat through. Add the anchovies, sage, breadcrumbs, parsley and pepper to taste and cook gently until they are crisp, then spoon over the mullet. Finish with just a squeeze of lemon. Delicious eaten with red onion, cucumber and tomato salad, with perhaps a few capers thrown in.

AT THE FISHMONGER
Ask your fishmonger to scale, fillet and pinbone
2 x 200 g/7 oz red mullet.

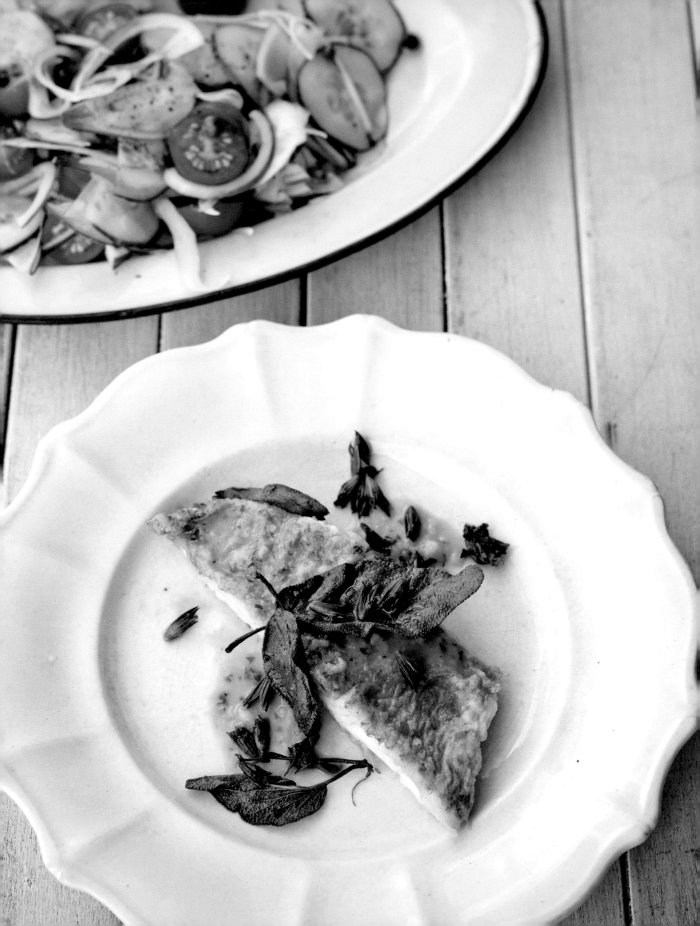

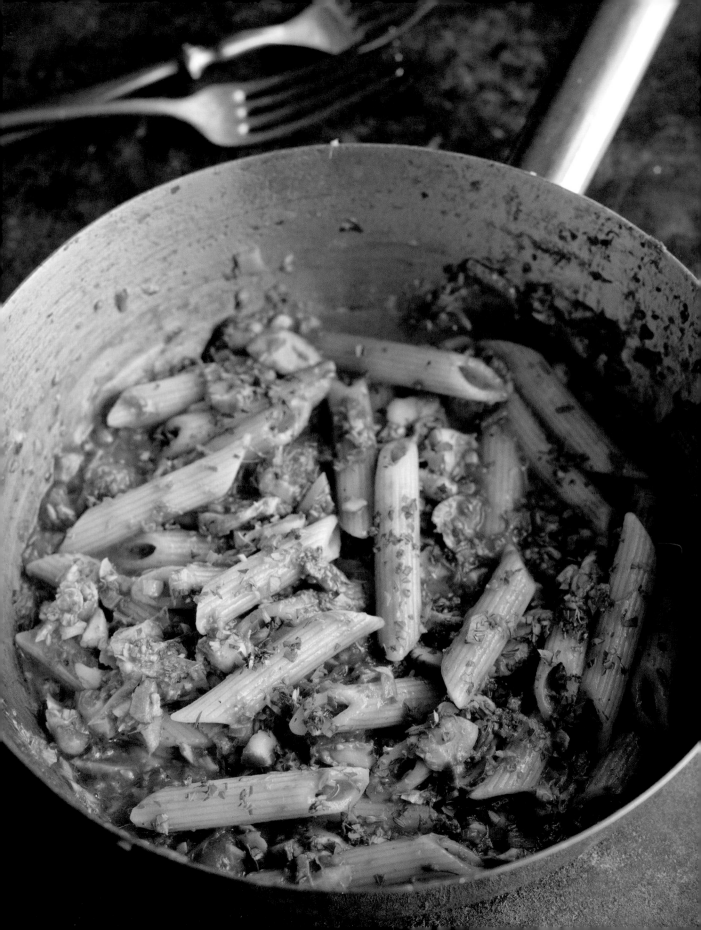

Red mullet is such a flavoursome fish and you can use small fillets in this recipe, which are very often cheaper, and plentiful in summer. I use red wine – and the dish is very rich, which makes it perfect to toss in pasta.

ragù of red mullet with penne

SERVES 4

extra virgin olive oil

1 garlic clove, finely chopped

1 tbsp very finely chopped celery

1 tbsp very finely chopped fennel

1 tbsp tomato purée

125 ml/4½ fl oz/generous ½ cup red wine

50 ml/2 fl oz/4 tbsp orange juice

6 ripe cherry tomatoes

1 star anise

½ tsp ground fennel seeds

piece of dried orange peel

pinch of dried oregano

3 small red mullet (or red snapper), scaled, filleted and pinboned

150 g/5½ oz penne

small handful of fresh flat-leaf parsley, finely chopped

sea salt and freshly ground black pepper

Heat 2 tbsp olive oil in a pan and fry the garlic, celery and fennel gently until soft and lightly golden. Add the tomato purée and cook for 3–4 minutes, then add the red wine, increase the heat and boil to reduce by at least half. Add the orange juice and boil until reduced by half again, then add the whole cherry tomatoes, star anise, ground fennel, orange peel and oregano. Lay the fish fillets in the pan and cover. Reduce the heat to medium-low and simmer for 15 minutes, then stir to break up the fish. Remove the orange peel and star anise.

Meanwhile, boil the penne in a large pan of lightly salted boiling water until al dente, then strain and add to the sauce, using a little of the cooking water if necessary to loosen the sauce, which should lightly cling to the pasta. Sprinkle with chopped parsley, season and serve.

AT THE FISHMONGER
Ask your fishmonger to scale, fillet and pinbone 3 small red mullet.

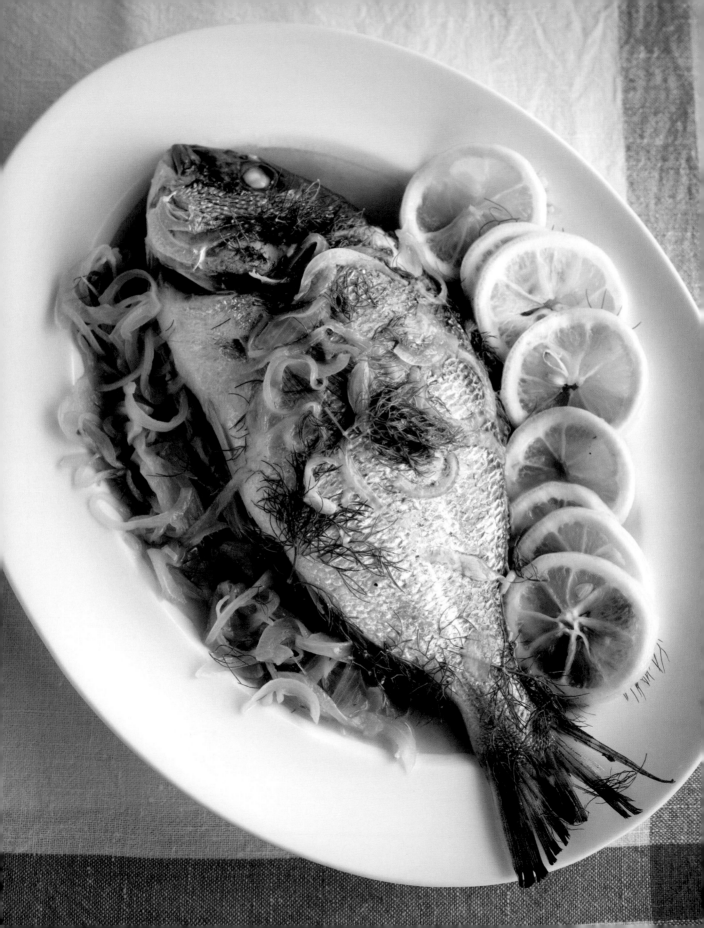

Wild fennel and wet (new-season) garlic are about at the same time, so I tend to use them together, but this dish works just as well with a fennel bulb and ordinary garlic, so don't be put off. I like to eat my fish from the bone, but if you don't, just use fillets and shorten the cooking time by about 6 minutes.

sea bream with wild fennel and garlic

SERVES 2

1 head of new-season garlic, sliced thinly from top to bottom

1 onion, thinly sliced

2 tbsp olive oil

1 tbsp Pernod or pastis

2 sea bream, each 450 g/ 1 lb, scaled, gutted and fins removed

1 lemon, thinly sliced

a few branches of wild fennel

25 g/1 oz/2 tbsp butter

sea salt and freshly ground black pepper

a little lemon juice (optional)

In a lidded frying pan big enough to take the fish, gently cook the garlic and onion in the olive oil until golden. Add the Pernod or pastis and increase the heat to boil off some of the alcohol, then lay the fish on top and cover each one with lemon slices and a sprinkling of wild fennel. Cover and simmer very gently over a low heat for 12 minutes, so that the fish is steaming in the pan. If it looks like it needs moisture, add a little water.

Remove the fish, onion, garlic and lemon, then whisk the butter into the pan juices, taste and season. Add a little lemon juice if needed. Lay the fish on a plate, pour over the sauce and put the onions and fennel on top.

AT THE FISHMONGER
Ask your fishmonger to scale, gut and trim the fins from 2 x 450 g/1 lb sea bream.

sea bass with clams and sherry

SERVES 2

A very simple one-pot dish. Fry **1 whole garlic clove** in **a little olive oil** over a medium-high heat until it starts to brown, then place **2 sea bass fillets** in the pan, skin side down, and cook over a high heat until they brown – 4–5 minutes. Turn them over, add **10–15 clams** (ensure they are closed or close when tapped sharply and the shells aren't damaged), **2 chopped cherry tomatoes** and **100 ml/3½ fl oz/½ cup dry sherry**, then cover and cook for a further 5 minutes, until the clams are open (discard any that remain closed). The bass should be just cooked by now too, so add a **handful of fresh coriander leaves** (cilantro), season to taste with **sea salt** and serve.

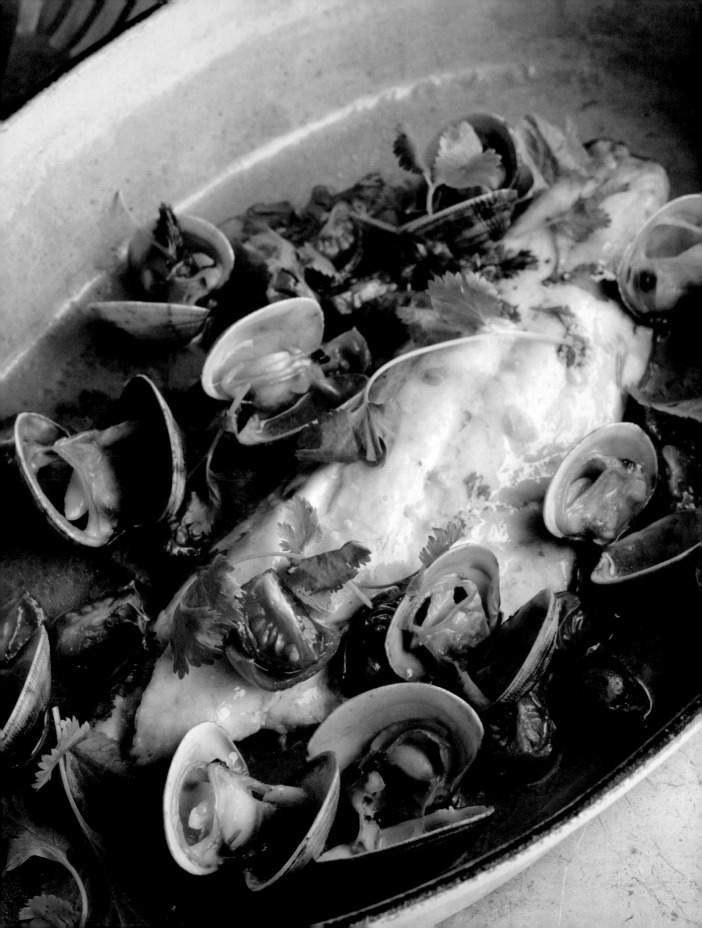

The mass production of salmon puts a few people off eating it, but it is still one of our most popular fish. I like a piece of poached salmon; the moistness it offers is all part of the enjoyment of this fish. I particularly like to eat the wild fish once a year, as a treat to mark springtime. However, I often make this dish as a quick lunch with reared fish, which I have no aversion to if it is from the right producer (for instance Loch Duart, Glenarm or Clare Island).

poached salmon with cucumber and dill mayonnaise

SERVES 4

1 chunk of salmon, cut from the middle of the fish, about 750 g/ 1 lb 10 oz

75 ml/2½ fl oz/5 tbsp dry white wine

juice of ½ lemon

a few peppercorns

a few parsley or tarragon stalks

sea salt and freshly ground black pepper

250 ml/9 fl oz/generous 1 cup mayonnaise (shop bought, or use the easy recipe on page 195)

3–4 tbsp finely chopped cucumber

1 tbsp finely chopped fresh dill

1 tbsp salted capers, rinsed and chopped

lightly dressed watercress to serve

Place the salmon in a pan, add the wine, lemon, peppercorns, parsley or tarragon stalks and a pinch of salt. Cover with water, bring gently to the boil, then simmer for about 5 minutes. Turn off the heat, cover the pan and leave for a further 30 minutes to allow the residual heat to cook the fish.

Mix the mayonnaise with the cucumber, dill and capers and season to taste.

Remove the fish from the water, then peel off the skin. Carve the fish into nice chunks, removing any bones, then season and serve with lightly dressed watercress and the cucumber and dill mayonnaise.

A very quick supper dish full of Mediterranean flavours. Because monkfish is so firm, it's perfect for stewing. A handful of clams or mussels thrown in at the end is a nice addition.

monkfish, caper and olive stew

SERVES 2

6 ripe tomatoes

4 tbsp olive oil

2 slices of monkfish cut across the tail, each 200 g/7 oz, skin and membrane removed

1 garlic clove, finely chopped

1 onion, thinly sliced

175 ml/6 fl oz/¾ cup dry white wine

10 black olives, pitted

1 tbsp salted capers, rinsed

10 fresh basil leaves

juice of 1 lemon

sea salt

To skin the tomatoes, pierce them with a knife, then drop them into a bowl of just-boiled water for 2 minutes. Remove from the bowl with a spoon, leave to cool for a few seconds, then peel off the skins. Roughly chop the flesh.

Heat the olive oil in a pan over a medium-high heat and sear the monkfish until golden on each side, then remove from the pan and set aside, covered. Reduce the heat to medium. Add the garlic and onion and cook for 8–10 minutes until the onion is softened. Add the wine and boil off the alcohol – this will take a minute. Add the chopped tomatoes and stir.

Place the fish back in the pan with the olives and capers, cover and simmer for 10 minutes, until cooked. Stir in the basil and lemon juice, season to taste with sea salt and serve.

AT THE FISHMONGER
Ask your fishmonger to remove the skin and membrane from a piece of monkfish, about 400 g/14 oz.

Red mullet has particular qualities that make the flavour very rich. The secret of this soup is making a good stock. Additionally, you want just a flicker of movement on it as it develops on the stove top; if you let it do its own thing it eventually comes together to produce delightful results. I also use this as a base to cook fish, fennel and potatoes and serve them in a clay pot as a more robust fish stew. It takes some time to cook, but just minutes to prepare.

red mullet soup

SERVES 4

1 fennel bulb, finely chopped

2 celery sticks (stalks), finely chopped

4 garlic cloves, finely chopped

2 tbsp olive oil

150 ml/5 fl oz/⅔ cup dry white wine

2 x 400 g/14 oz cans tomatoes

10 salted anchovy fillets

4 litres/7 pints/4 quarts shellfish stock (see page 208)

1 tbsp fennel seeds

good pinch of saffron strands

3 bay leaves

sprig of fresh thyme

6 red mullet, scaled, filleted and pinboned

saffron mayonnaise (see page 202), finely chopped curly parsley and fried bread to serve

Gently fry the fennel, celery and garlic in the olive oil over a medium heat until lightly golden and soft – 4–5 minutes. Add the wine, boil off the alcohol, then add the tomatoes, anchovies, stock, fennel seeds and saffron. Using a hand blender, blend the liquid until smooth, then pour into a large pan. Add the bay and thyme and bring to the boil, then reduce the heat and simmer very lightly – you just want a flicker of movement – uncovered, for 1½ hours.

Add the mullet fillets, then simmer very gently, uncovered, for 2 hours until the flavour has developed and the mullet is broken up. Taste it often – you will know when it is ready. Serve with saffron mayonnaise, a sprinkle of parsley and some fried bread.

AT THE FISHMONGER
Ask your fishmonger to scale, fillet and pinbone 6 red mullet.

This is a delicious sauce that requires loads of wild fennel. I harvest a lot of it in early summer and blitz the fronds, then keep them in oil for dishes like this and for marinades. I use the dried stalks for our grill at my restaurant The Seahorse. This dish has a lovely balance of flavours – strong sardines, salty anchovies, heady fennel and sweet raisins and onion.

bucatini with sardines, chard and wild fennel

SERVES 4

2 (Swiss) chard, leaves and stalks separated

sea salt

olive oil

1 large onion, thinly sliced

1 tsp anchovy paste

1 tbsp good-quality raisins, soaked in warm water for 15 minutes and drained

8 sardines, scaled, filleted, pinboned and roughly chopped

100 ml/3½ fl oz/½ cup good tomato sauce or passata (strained tomatoes, not tomato paste)

large handful of wild fennel fronds, plus extra to serve

1 garlic clove, grated

150 g/5½ oz bucatini (or you can use macaroni)

1 tbsp pine nuts

extra virgin olive oil and lemon wedges to serve

Cook the chard leaves in a little lightly salted boiling water for 2 minutes, then drain and squeeze dry. Blanch the stalks for 3–4 minutes in a separate pan. Drain and set aside.

Heat 2 tbsp olive oil in a pan, then gently cook the onion for 8 minutes until softened and golden. Add the anchovy paste, raisins, sardines and tomato sauce or passata and stew for a few minutes. Add the fennel and a little water if the mixture seems too dry, then cover and stew gently for 10 minutes until it has all cooked down into a thick sauce.

In another pan, lightly brown the garlic in olive oil, then add the chard stems and leaves and the sauce. Cook the bucatini as on the packet instructions, then strain and add to the chard pan with a little of the cooking water. Serve sprinkled with fennel fronds, pine nuts and a drizzle of very good olive oil, with lemon wedges on the side.

AT THE FISHMONGER
Ask your fishmonger to scale, fillet and pinbone 8 sardines.

I don't usually like fried oily fish, but here the batter is extremely light and works very well. This recipe is also good made with small gurnard fillets.

sardine fritters with caper mayonnaise

SERVES 4

2 large eggs, separated

200 g/7 oz/1 cup plain (all-purpose) flour

sea salt and freshly ground black pepper

vegetable oil for deep-frying

8 sardines, scaled, filleted and pinboned (tails left on)

75 g/2½ oz/½ cup salted capers, drained and roughly chopped

200 ml/7 fl oz/scant 1 cup mayonnaise (see page 195)

lemon wedges to serve

Make the batter 1 hour before cooking. Beat the egg yolks and mix with the flour and salt to taste and enough water to make a thick batter (about the consistency of double/heavy cream). Season well with black pepper. Whisk the egg whites until stiff peaks form, then fold into the batter.

Half fill a deep-fat fryer with vegetable oil and heat to 190°C/375°F, or until a cube of bread browns in 30 seconds.

Dry each sardine fillet well, then dip in the batter. Fry until puffed and crisp – 3–4 minutes.

Add the capers to the mayonnaise and serve alongside the fritters, with lemon wedges.

AT THE FISHMONGER
Ask your fishmonger to scale, fillet and pinbone 8 sardines.

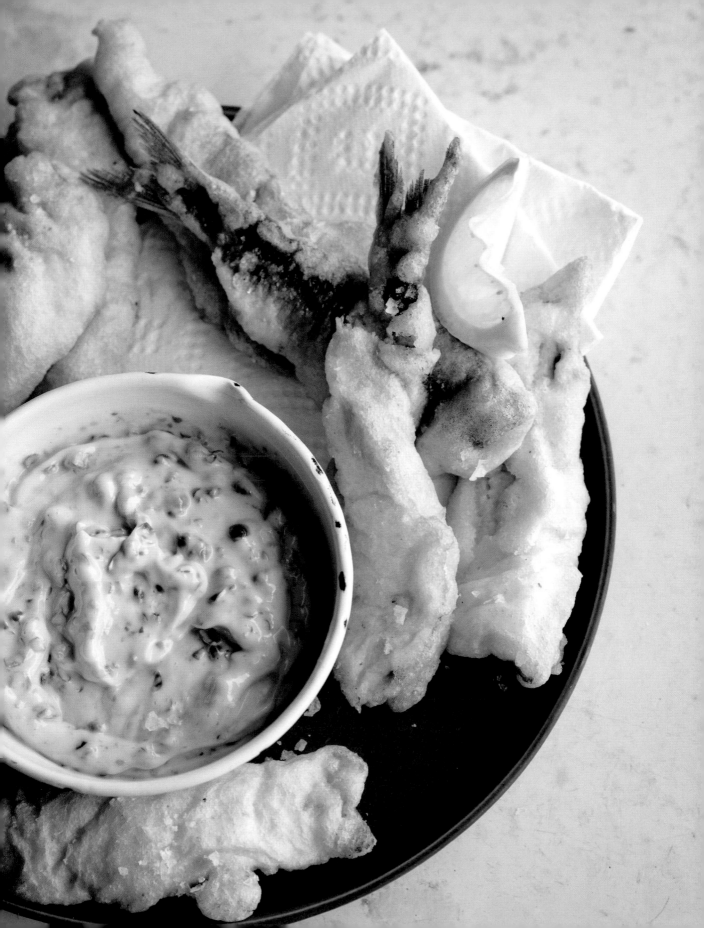

herring roe pâté

SERVES 2

A delicious savoury pâté, wonderful spread on thick hot toast. Soak 200 g/7 oz herring milts (or roes) in milk for 1 hour. Drain and dry, then fry in a little butter until just firmed up and cooked. Add the contents of the pan to a food processor with a further spoonful of soft butter, a pinch of mustard or curry powder, a few rinsed salted capers and 2 salted anchovy fillets. Blitz until smooth, then spoon into a small dish, cover and put in the fridge to set; you can, if you wish, top with clarified butter.

I love sardine paste sandwiches with thinly sliced cucumber. I often catch a glut of mackerel at home in Brixham and make this paste as a way of using them up.

mackerel paste

MAKES 1 X 250 ML/9 FL OZ JAR

4 medium mackerel, gutted, deheaded and tails removed

1 onion, thinly sliced

sprig of fresh thyme

2 tbsp white wine vinegar

1 tbsp good tomato purée (you can make your own by cooking skinned and seeded tomatoes until well reduced, but a good shop-bought one will be fine)

handful of fresh dill

juice of ½ lemon

1 tsp horseradish sauce

a few cornichons (baby gherkins)

50 g/2 oz/4 tbsp crème fraîche (sour cream)

sea salt and freshly ground black pepper

In a pan large enough to take the mackerel, heat enough water to just cover them, then add the fish, onion, thyme and vinegar. Bring to the boil, then take off the heat and allow the fish to cool in the water, where it will finish cooking.

Lift the mackerel out of the water, then remove all the skin and flesh from the bones.

Place the fish, tomato paste, dill, lemon juice, horseradish and cornichons in a food processor and blitz to a smooth paste. Stir in the crème fraîche and salt and freshly ground black pepper to taste, then spoon into a pot and chill.

AT THE FISHMONGER
Ask your fishmonger to gut, top and tail 4 medium mackerel.

Hot, salty and sweet, with fresh mint and coriander leaves, this really is a great combination.

Vietnamese-style fried squid

SERVES 4

500 g/1 lb 2 oz cleaned and prepared squid (calamari), cut into rings

1 tbsp vegetable oil

1 garlic clove, crushed to a paste

1 red chilli (chile), deseeded and finely chopped

small handful of fresh mint, finely chopped

small handful of fresh coriander (cilantro), finely chopped

For the sauce
1 red chilli (chile), deseeded and chopped

2 garlic cloves, crushed to a paste

100 ml/3½ fl oz/½ cup fish sauce

3 tbsp caster (superfine) sugar

50 ml/2 fl oz/4 tbsp white wine vinegar

juice of 1 lime

Combine the sauce ingredients in a bowl, then add the squid, cover and leave to marinate in the fridge for 1 hour.

Heat the vegetable oil in a wok or pan, then add the garlic and chilli. When the garlic starts to brown, add the squid and stir-fry for 4–5 minutes. Add any remaining marinade, simmer for a few minutes, then stir in the mint and coriander and serve.

AT THE FISHMONGER
Ask your fishmonger to clean and skin the squid.

Fried squid (calamari) needs to be crisp. The simplest coating of all is milk and flour, and this works perfectly for me. Try to buy small squid with pure white flesh and no signs of pinkness.

fried squid with chilli-salt and pepper

SERVES 4 TO START

3 tbsp sea salt

2 tsp black peppercorns

2 tsp Sichuan peppercorns

4 small dried bird's-eye chillies (chiles)

small handful of '00' flour

small handful of cornflour (cornstarch)

300 ml/10 fl oz/1¼ cups milk

vegetable oil for deep-frying

350 g/12 oz cleaned and prepared squid (calamari), cut into rings

small handful of fresh coriander (cilantro) leaves, roughly chopped

lime wedges to serve

Mix the salt and peppercorns together, then roast them in a dry pan over a medium-high heat for a few minutes, until really fragrant. Leave to cool, then tip them into a pestle and mortar, add the dried chillies and grind finely. Mix two-thirds of this with the flour and cornflour in a shallow bowl. Put the milk in a second shallow bowl.

Half fill a deep-fat fryer or wok with vegetable oil and heat to 190°C/375°F, or until a cube of bread browns in 30 seconds. Dip the squid in the milk, then in the flour mixture. Carefully lower each piece into the fryer and fry until light in colour and crisp – 3–4 minutes.

To serve, sprinkle with the remaining salt, pepper and chilli mix and scatter with coriander. Serve the lime wedges on the side.

AT THE FISHMONGER
Ask your fishmonger to clean and skin the squid.

in the pan

It's a mystery to me why cuttlefish hasn't enjoyed the popularity in England that it has in Italy and Spain, where most of it is sent after it has been landed by British fishermen. Cuttlefish has a good flavour (better than squid, which is much more popular, and it's about a quarter of the price).

spaghetti with cuttlefish and ink sauce

SERVES 2

olive oil

2 cloves garlic, finely chopped

1 small onion, finely chopped

1 kg/2 lb 4 oz cleaned and prepared cuttlefish, cut into strips

sea salt and freshly ground black pepper

75 ml/2½ fl oz/⅓ cup dry white wine

3 tbsp tomato purée

8 tomatoes, roughly chopped

small handful of curly parsley, finely chopped

2 tbsp cuttlefish or squid ink

200 g/7 oz spaghetti

Pour a generous glug of olive oil into a casserole dish over a medium heat. Add the garlic and onion and fry for 5–6 minutes, until lightly golden. Add the cuttlefish and fry for a further 1–2 minutes. Season with salt, then pour in the wine and cook until it has reduced by half.

Add the tomato purée, tomatoes and a little more wine or water if the pan is too dry (the cuttlefish will release liquid as it cooks) and cook for another minute. Add half the parsley and lastly all the ink, stir, bring to a gentle simmer, cover and cook gently for about 45–50 minutes, until the cuttlefish is really tender when you stick a knife into it (it should have the texture of braised belly pork fat; if you need to cook it longer to get there then do so).

If you have lots of liquid still in the pan, ladle most of it out into another saucepan and boil to reduce it by as much as you need to thicken it, then add it back to the stew. The final texture should be thick, so that when you spoon it on to plates you don't have juice spilling out of it.

Meanwhile, boil the spaghetti until al dente, then drain. Add it to the cuttlefish sauce. Serve sprinkled with the remaining parsley.

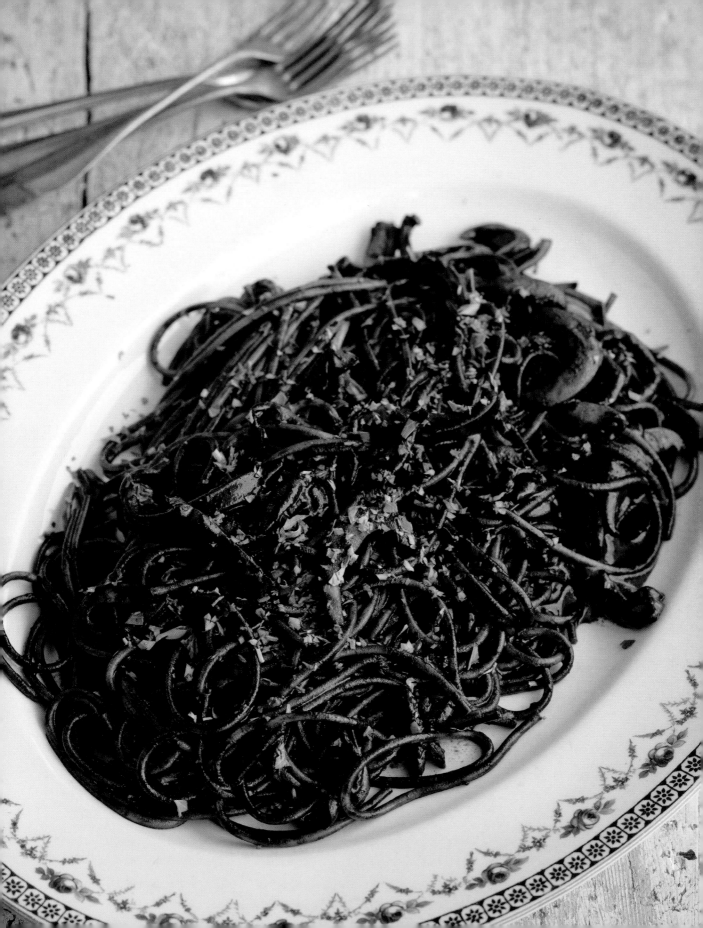

I'm a big fan of cuttlefish; it looks daunting when whole, but after the fishmonger has done the preparation, you are left with pure white meat. This dish works well with squid (calamari) too. I keep a few packs of frozen peas, broad (fava) beans and artichoke hearts handy, but very early in the summer, when everything is young and new, make this with fresh vegetables.

cuttlefish with summer vegetables, mint and aioli

SERVES 4

700 g/1 lb 9oz cleaned and prepared cuttlefish

2 tbsp olive oil

2 garlic cloves, finely chopped

1 tbsp dry white wine

sprig of fresh tarragon

150 ml/5 fl oz/⅔ cup good chicken or vegetable stock

4 small violet artichokes, prepared and quartered, then cooked until soft

handful of blanched and skinned broad (fava) beans

handful of peas

sea salt and freshly ground black pepper

squeeze of lemon juice

1 tbsp finely chopped fresh mint

5 tbsp mayonnaise (see page 195)

Using the tip of a sharp knife, slice the cuttlefish from top to bottom, then open it out and make diagonal cuts, first one way and then the other, on the inside, making sure the depth of the cut is just halfway through the thickness. Then cut into strips about 2.5 cm/1 in x 7.5 cm/3 in.

Heat the olive oil in a pan over a high heat. Add half the garlic, then all the cuttlefish, and stir-fry for 1 minute – it should curl up on itself. Add the wine and boil for a minute or two to reduce, then reduce the heat to low-medium, add the tarragon and simmer very gently – you will see plenty of juice coming out of the cuttlefish, but if it looks dry just add a splash of water. Cook the cuttlefish like this for about 40 minutes, until it is white and tender, then lift it out of the liquid and set aside.

Warm the stock in a separate pan, add the vegetables and simmer until softened – 5 minutes. Add the cuttlefish and season.

For the aioli, mix a little lemon juice, the mint and remaining garlic into the mayonnaise in a pestle and mortar and really work it until thoroughly combined. Serve the stew in bowls with the aioli on the side to stir in.

AT THE FISHMONGER

Ask your fishmonger to clean 700 g/1 lb 9 oz cuttlefish, making sure no membrane or black residue from the ink remains.

Frozen, skinned baby onions are perfect for this dish. Use frozen, fresh, jarred or canned Spanish branded peas; all of them have different qualities and are equally delicious. My preference is for the bottled Spanish ones, their sweetness is wonderful with the squid (calamari).

squid with pearl onions, peas and parsley

SERVES 4

350 g/12 oz cleaned and prepared squid (calamari)

2 tbsp olive oil

150 g/5½ oz frozen skinned baby onions

2 garlic cloves, finely chopped

50 ml/2 fl oz/4 tbsp dry white wine

100 ml/3½ fl oz/½ cup good chicken stock

200 g/7 oz peas (see introduction)

sea salt and freshly ground black pepper

juice of ½ lemon

small handful of fresh flat-leaf parsley, finely chopped

Slice the squid from top to bottom, then open it out and make diagonal cuts across the squid first one way and then the other, making sure the depth of the cut is just halfway through the thickness. Cut the squid lengthways from the top of the squid to the bottom into strips about 2.5 cm/1 in wide.

Heat the olive oil in a pan and gently cook the whole frozen onions until starting to turn golden, then add the garlic. When this starts to brown, increase the heat to high, add the squid and sauté, vigorously moving it around the hot pan, for 4–5 minutes. Add the wine and wait for it to sizzle and boil away, then add the stock and peas and cook gently for 1 minute to allow them to warm through. Season, squeeze in the lemon juice and serve sprinkled with the parsley.

AT THE FISHMONGER
Ask your fishmonger to clean and skin 350 g/12 oz squid.

This is a wonderful dish that I first ate in Café Belear in Menorca. They served it in a big chunky clay pot, the *caldereta*; I can still taste it to this day. My version is a favourite at my restaurant The Seahorse.

braised lobster with sherry and onions

SERVES 4

1 live lobster, about 650 g/1 lb 7 oz

2 tbsp olive oil

2 onions, thinly sliced

3 garlic cloves, finely chopped

1 bay leaf

100 ml/3½ fl oz/½ cup manzanilla sherry

sea salt and freshly ground black pepper

1 tbsp finely chopped fresh flat-leaf parsley

Place the lobster on a chopping board. Insert a large, sharp, heavy knife into the cross on the back of the head and cut down towards the tail, cutting it in half. Remove the stomach and the black intestinal tract (if there is one) that may run through the middle of the tail and discard. Cut the lobster into chunks.

Heat the olive oil in a pan over a gentle heat. Cook the lobster chunks for 6–7 minutes, then remove and set aside. Add the onions and garlic to the pan, then cover and cook slowly over a low heat for about 40 minutes – the secret of this dish is the very slow cooking of the onions, to almost caramelize but not brown them.

Return the lobster chunks to the pan and add the bay leaf, then cover and cook gently for 2–3 minutes. Add the sherry and simmer for a further 5 minutes. Check the seasoning. Pour into a warm casserole dish, sprinkle with the parsley and put into the centre of the table for everyone to help themselves.

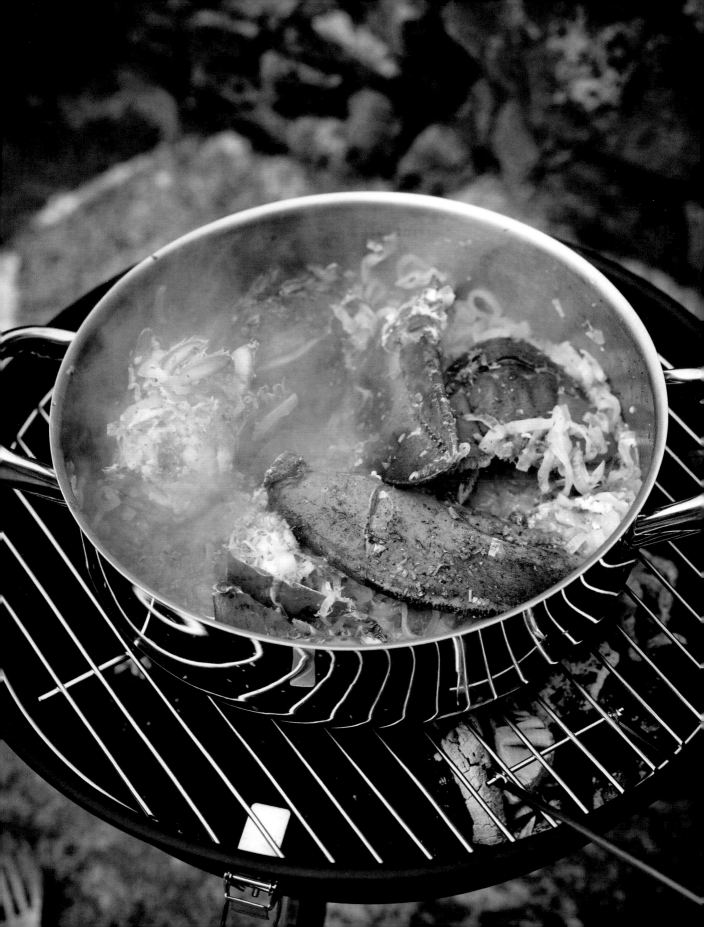

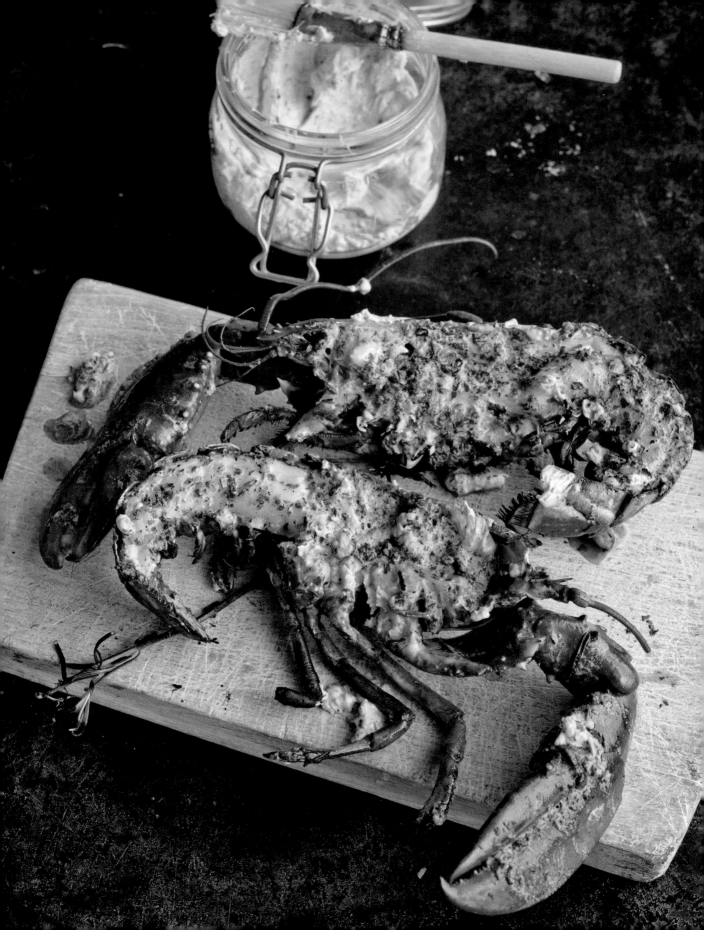

I've always been a big fan of grilled and roasted lobster. Recently, in our RockFish restaurant, we have been serving lobsters freshly steamed with melted butter and I love them cooked this way now. It's very easy to do and if you have friends coming round, cover the table in newspaper, steam a few lobsters (as many as you can afford), pop them in the middle of the table and serve with this melted butter and herb sauce.

steamed lobster with herb butter sauce

SERVES 4

4 live lobsters, about 650 g/1 lb 7 oz each

a few handfuls of edible seaweed

sea salt (optional)

1 tbsp old bay-style seasoning (optional), made by grinding together 1 tsp celery seeds, pinch of mace, 2 cardamom pods, ½ tsp mustard seeds, 4 cloves, pinch of paprika, pinch of ginger, 1 tsp black peppercorns and 4 bay leaves

250 g/9 oz/generous 1 cup salted butter

3 egg yolks

pinch of cayenne pepper

juice of 1 lemon

1 tbsp finely chopped fresh chervil

1 tbsp finely chopped fresh chives

1 tbsp finely chopped fresh curly parsley

good waxy potatoes, freshly boiled, to serve

Place the lobster on a chopping board. Insert a large, sharp, heavy knife into the cross on the back of the head to kill it.

Steam the lobsters just before you serve them, so they are still warm on the table. To do this, pour 600 ml/20 fl oz/2½ cups or so of water into a large pan, bring to the boil, then add the seaweed, a few tbsp salt and the old bay seasoning, if using. Add the lobsters (they should sit on the seaweed above the water), then cover and allow them to steam in the vapours for 15 minutes, keeping the water boiling. Transfer to a serving platter. Cut the lobsters in half; you will sometimes see a black vein running through the tail on one side – this is the intestinal tract and if the lobster has been digesting it will be prominent. Don't worry, it's not dangerous; simply flick it out with the tip of a knife.

Meanwhile, clarify the butter. Heat it gently in a saucepan until it melts. Remove from the heat. Slowly and carefully spoon the white froth off the butter – this takes patience. You should be left with only the yellow liquid butter.

To make the sauce, whisk the egg yolks with 1 tsp water in a pan over a gentle heat until smooth and light – do not scramble the eggs, just thicken them. Whisking continuously, slowly pour in the clarified butter until the sauce is thickened. Add the cayenne, lemon and herbs and serve with the hot lobster and potatoes.

A huge favourite at my restaurants The Seahorse and RockFish. I'm not a fan of cream with mussels – just their own juices and a splash of wine is good for me. Try mussels from different sources and you'll be amazed at how different they taste, depending on the environment from which they are harvested. I prefer those grown at sea, with small shells and big silky meats.

mussels with chilli, wine and bay leaves

SERVES 2 TO START

700 g/1 lb 9 oz mussels
good knob of butter
1 tbsp olive oil
1 shallot, finely chopped
1 garlic clove, finely chopped
handful of fresh curly parsley, finely chopped
2 bay leaves
2 small dried chillies (chiles)
75 ml/3 fl oz/5 tbsp dry white wine
sea salt and freshly ground black pepper
grilled or fried crusty bread to serve

Scrub the mussels and remove the wispy beards. Discard any shells that are broken or that are open and do not close when sharply tapped.

Heat the butter and olive oil in a pan over a low-medium heat, add the shallot and garlic and cook for 4–5 minutes to soften. Add the parsley and bay leaves and crumble in the chillies. Add the mussels and toss in the pan to coat the shells well, then add the wine, cover and cook for 3–4 minutes to allow the mussels to steam open (discard any that remain closed).

Season with salt and pepper, then pour into a bowl and serve with grilled or fried crusty bread.

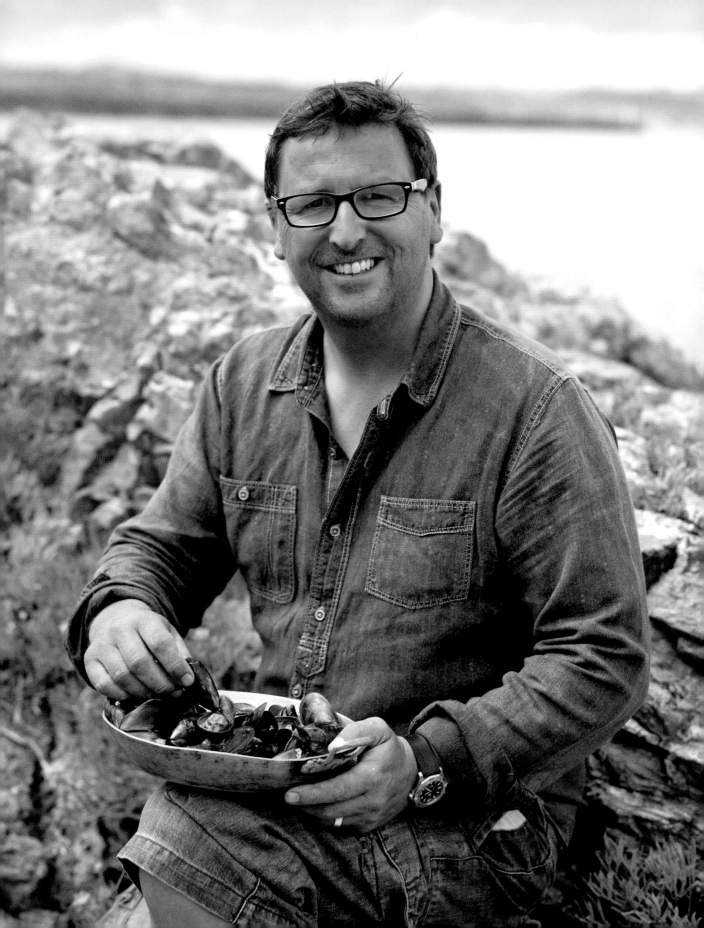

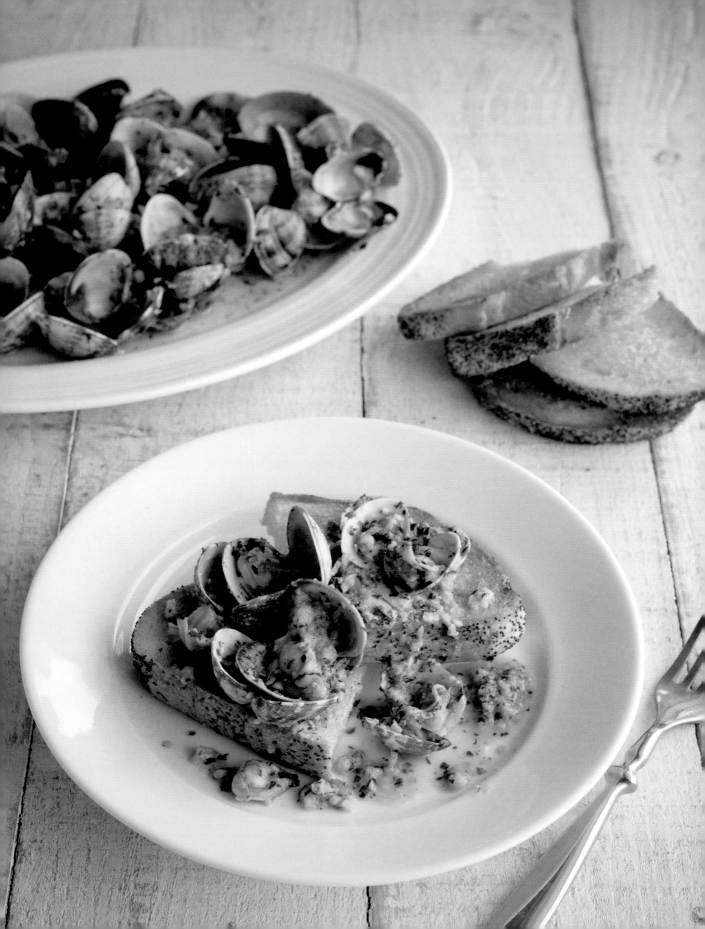

When I see a dish that has 'marinara' or 'fisherman' in the title I'm drawn to it; I usually think it's what the guys in the know eat, and often I'm right. There's nothing clever about this simple preparation, the breadcrumbs just soak up the juices and somehow the combination of parsley, garlic, anchovies and just a little wine do really taste of the sea.

sailors' clams

SERVES 4 TO START

1 kg/2 lb 4 oz clams

olive oil

1 garlic clove, finely chopped, plus
1 whole clove

75 ml/2½ fl oz/5 tbsp dry white wine

2 or 3 salted anchovies

handful of fresh curly parsley

handful of fine fresh breadcrumbs

freshly ground black pepper
(optional)

bread to serve

Wash the clams and discard any shells that are broken or that are open and do not close when sharply tapped.

Warm 2 tbsp olive oil in a frying pan over a medium-high heat. Add the chopped garlic and cook until it just starts to brown, then add the clams and give the pan a good toss to get them coated with the garlic and oil. Add the wine and anchovies, cover the pan and boil for 3–4 minutes, or until the clams are open (discard any that remain closed).

Chop the parsley finely with the whole garlic clove and mix with the breadcrumbs. Fry in a separate pan with a little oil until just crisp, then gradually sprinkle them into the clams until the sauce thickens slightly. Add some pepper, if you like, then serve over slices of yesterday's bread or with fried bread.

A seafood stew is much quicker to cook than a meat stew. I've used Marsala wine in this recipe, which is inspired by a prawn dish that I ate in Sicily. You can use any shellfish for this dish; I've included lobster here but you can leave that out if you wish and stir in a couple of tablespoons of white crab meat at the last minute instead. Frozen peas are also delicious if broad (fava) beans aren't available.

shellfish stew with broad beans and savory

SERVES 4

500 g/1 lb 2 oz mussels

500 g/1 lb 2 oz clams

500 g/1 lb 2 oz cockles

1 live lobster, about 650 g/1 lb 7 oz

50 ml/2 fl oz/4 tbsp dry white wine

50 ml/2 fl oz/4 tbsp olive oil

4 garlic cloves

20 raw prawns, peeled and deveined – keep the shells

50 ml/2 fl oz/4 tbsp Marsala

50–60 ml/2–2½ fl oz/4 tbsp double (heavy) cream

small handful of savory leaves

1 small dried chilli (chile), crumbled

150 g/5½ oz broad (fava) beans, blanched and skinned

handful of fresh flat-leaf parsley, finely chopped

lemon wedges to serve

Scrub the mussels and remove the wispy beards. Wash the clams and cockles. Discard any shells that are broken or that are open and do not close when sharply tapped.

Bring a large saucepan of water to the boil, then add the lobster and blanch for 5 minutes. Remove from the pan and extract the meat from the shell. Reserve the shell and chop into pieces.

Put the mussels, clams and cockles in a saucepan with the wine, cover the pan and boil for 3–4 minutes until they all open. Discard any that remain closed. Remove the rest from the shells and reserve, then strain the juices and reserve these too.

Heat the olive oil in a large frying pan, add the garlic and cook over a medium heat until it starts to brown. Add the reserved lobster shells and the prawn shells and fry for 5–8 minutes – this gives the oil in the pan a lovely richness – then strain off the oil, discard the shells and garlic and return the oil to the pan.

Add the lobster meat and prawns and fry over a high heat for 3–4 minutes. Add the Marsala and cook for 2–3 minutes to boil off the alcohol, then add the reserved juices from the molluscs and boil down by half. Reduce the heat, add the cream, savory, chilli, mussels, clams, cockles and broad beans and simmer for a further 3–4 minutes, until thickened and warmed through. Sprinkle with parsley and serve with lemon wedges.

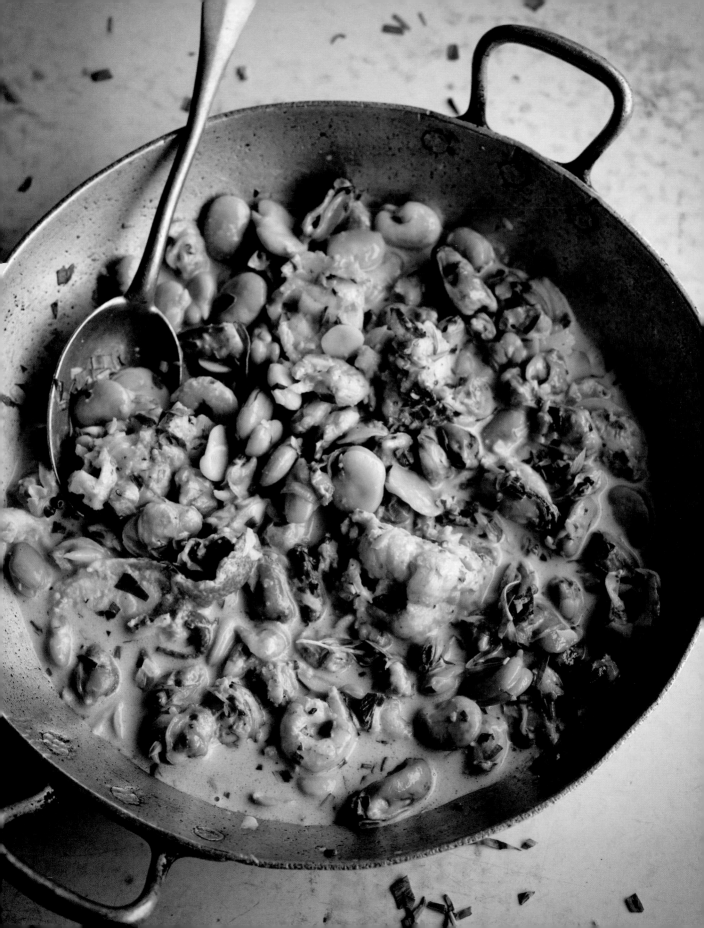

clams and peas with sherry and coriander

SERVES 1

Wash **300 g/10½ oz clams** and discard any shells that are damaged or that are open and do not close when sharply tapped. Gently fry **2 finely chopped garlic cloves** in **olive oil** over a low heat until golden. Add the clams and then **100 ml/ 3½ fl oz/½ cup dry sherry** (manzanilla or fino). Cover and allow the clams to steam open (discard any that remain closed), then add **a handful of fresh or frozen peas** and cook for a few more minutes. Season with **freshly ground black pepper.** Finish with **a handful of chopped fresh coriander** (cilantro) and serve.

pan-roasted prawns in sticky chilli sauce

SERVES 2

For a quick and delicious supper, heat **2 tbsp olive oil**, add **a dozen tiger prawns** and sauté them gently until just turning orange. Add **4 tbsp nam jim sauce** (see page 38) and cook until the sauce is sticky and coating the prawns – 3–4 minutes. Serve with **lime wedges** and a sprinkling of **chopped fresh coriander (cilantro)**.

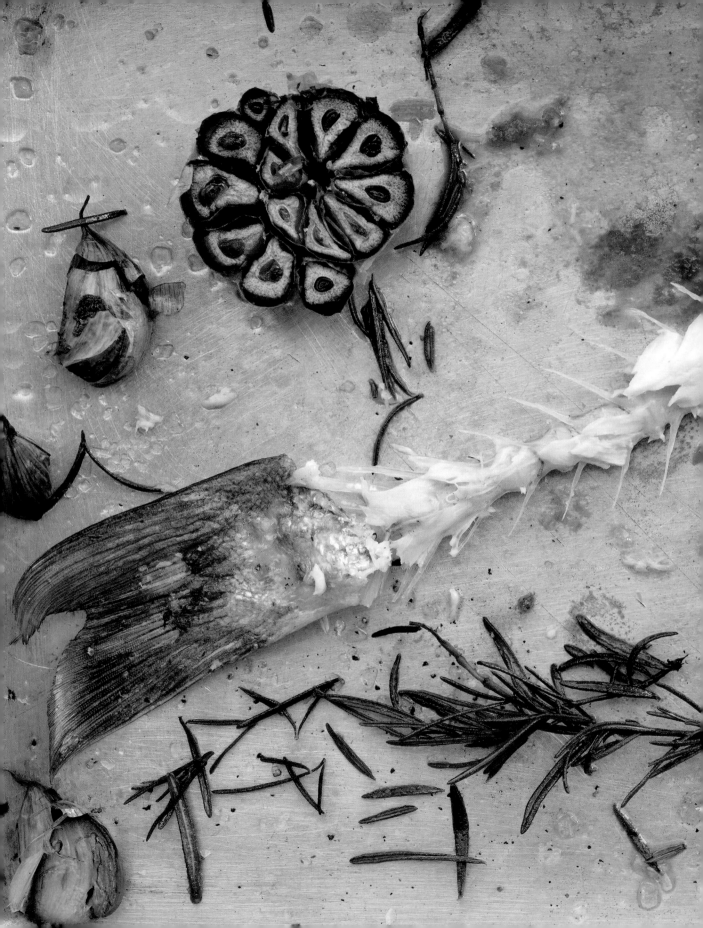

in the oven

roasting fish

Your oven offers by far the best method for cooking a fish that is larger than 450 g/1 lb. Roasting gives a fish crisp skin and moist flesh. You can add other ingredients to the dish to make a good sauce or accompaniment; for example, roasting a sea bass on top of part-cooked potatoes with plenty of oregano, lemon juice, wine and olive oil produces great results.

It is best to start by preheating the oven to maximum. Add a few glugs of good olive oil to a heavy roasting pan. Place some herbs inside your scaled and gutted fish (rosemary, sage, oregano and thyme work well), then put the fish in the roasting pan and season well with sea salt and freshly ground black pepper inside and out.

Now you can add your choice of accompaniments, such as cherry tomatoes, artichoke hearts, part-cooked potato wedges or slices, olives and capers. Roast at a high temperature – say 230°C/450°F/gas mark 8 – for about 5 minutes. Remove from the oven and add a small glass of dry white wine. Return to the oven and continue cooking for another 8 minutes or so. Remove again and sprinkle with fresh white breadcrumbs, then return to the oven until cooked. The breadcrumbs not only give a nice crispness to the dish, but also thicken the juices into a sauce.

When the fish is cooked, squeeze some lemon juice over it and add a sprinkling of fresh herbs. Serve it whole at the table, or take fillets from it. Serve the roasted vegetables alongside it and either spoon the juices over the top or serve them in a sauce boat.

I have eaten fish dishes like this – strong, salty, and sweet from ripe tomatoes – all over Sicily. I saw this made in one pan with loads of wine poured on; the fish simmered in the flavourings and served whole at the table, truly magnificent. If you can't get John Dory, try it with any fish.

John Dory with Messina sauce

SERVES 2

3 ripe tomatoes

extra virgin olive oil

2 garlic cloves, finely chopped

3 salted anchovy fillets

2 tbsp finely chopped fresh flat-leaf parsley

175 ml/6 fl oz/¾ cup dry white wine

1 tbsp tomato purée

1 tbsp salted capers, rinsed

10–15 small black olives, pitted

1 x 800–900 g/1 lb 12 oz–2 lb John Dory, scaled, gutted and fins trimmed off

small handful of fine fresh breadcrumbs

lemon wedges to serve

Preheat the oven to 240°C/475°F/gas mark 9. To skin the tomatoes, pierce them with a knife, then drop them into a bowl of just-boiled water for 2 minutes. Remove from the bowl with a spoon, leave to cool for a few seconds, then peel off the skins.

Pour a good glug of olive oil into a roasting pan large enough to take the fish. Place it over a medium heat and fry the garlic for 1–2 minutes, until it starts to brown. Add the anchovies and half the parsley, then immediately add the wine and boil for 1 minute.

Add the tomato purée, cook for 2 minutes, then squeeze in the skinned tomatoes. Add the capers and olives and stir well. Cook for 1–2 minutes more.

Move the mixture to one side of the dish, then lay the fish in the pan, spoon the mixture over the fish and bake for 15 minutes.

Baste the fish with the mixture and sprinkle with the breadcrumbs, then bake for a further 3–4 minutes, or until cooked through. Serve whole in the dish, nicely baked and crisp, sprinkled with the remaining parsley, with a few lemon wedges.

AT THE FISHMONGER
Ask your fishmonger to scale and gut a 800–900 g/ 1 lb 12 oz–2 lb John Dory and remove the fins.

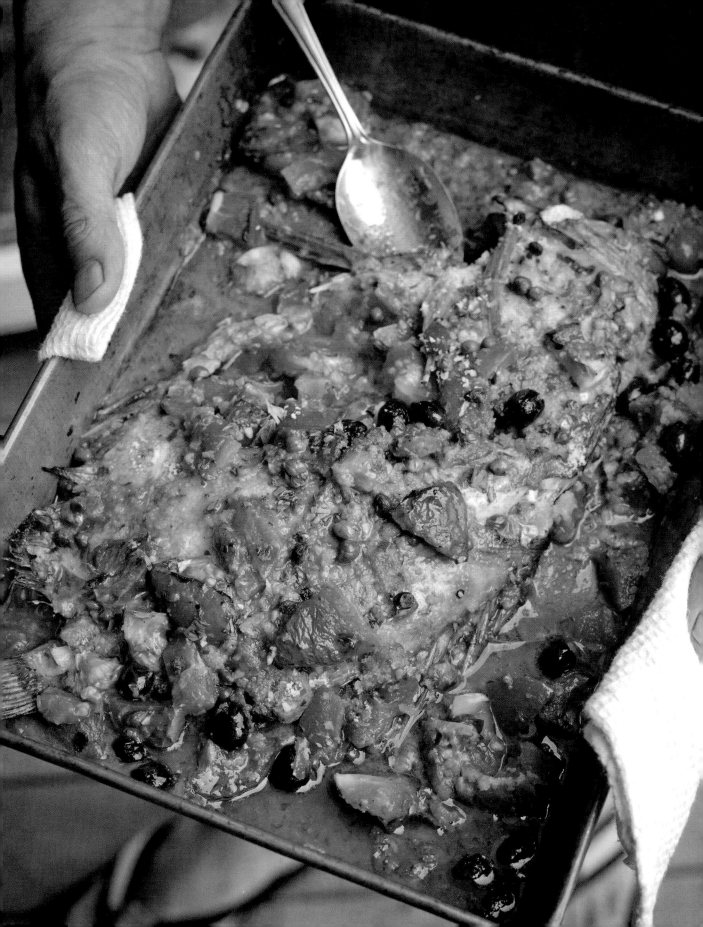

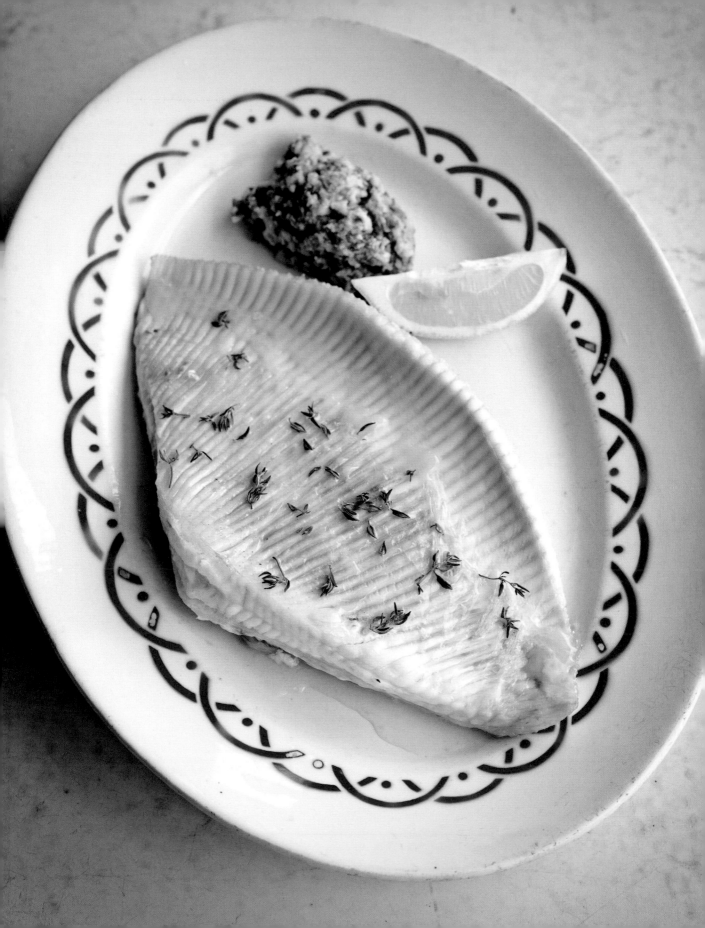

Most of the 'skate' we see these days is, in fact, a species of ray, but it is treated in the same way as skate. Here I roast it, but it is just as delicious lightly poached in water that has been flavoured with some aromatics – an onion, a carrot and a splash of wine. You don't get a crisp crust, but the flesh is softer. Leave it to cool and it is delicious in a salad. The sauce is very good with any simply grilled or roasted fish.

ray with herbs and capers

SERVES 2

2 tbsp vegetable oil

2 ray wings, each 350 g/12 oz, or slices from a larger fish

leaves from 2 sprigs of fresh thyme

lemon wedges to serve

For the salsa

a pinch of caster (superfine) sugar

100 ml/3½ fl oz/½ cup white wine vinegar

handful of fine fresh breadcrumbs

small handful of capers, roughly chopped (use salted capers if you can)

small handful of fresh flat-leaf parsley, finely chopped

small handful of chopped fresh basil

½ garlic clove, crushed

1 hard-boiled egg, white and yolk separated and finely grated

2 tbsp good olive oil

Preheat the oven to 240°C/475°F/gas mark 9. Heat the vegetable oil in a large ovenproof frying pan until hot. Dry the ray wings and place in the pan, thickest side down, then fry for 3–4 minutes. Add the thyme, then put in the oven for 8 minutes.

To make the salsa, dissolve the sugar in the vinegar, then soak the breadcrumbs in the vinegar mixture for 5 minutes. Mix in all the other ingredients.

Lift the fish from the pan – the underside should be crisp and golden – place on a plate and serve with the salsa, a sprinkling of rock salt and lemon wedges.

plaice with porcini, garlic and parsley

SERVES 1

Preheat the oven to 230°C/450°F/ gas mark 8.
Soak **a few dried porcini** in just-boiled water
for 15 minutes, then squeeze out the water.
Heat **1 tbsp olive oil** in an ovenproof frying
pan over a medium-high heat. Add **1 plaice
(or flounder) steak** (or you can use fillet) and
cook for 2–3 minutes on each side, then transfer
to the oven and cook for 6–8 minutes. Meanwhile,
melt **25 g/1 oz butter** in a pan over a medium-
low heat, add **1 finely chopped garlic clove**,
a handful of quartered **chestnut mushrooms**
and the **porcini** and **30 g/1 oz cooked spinach**.
Sauté for a few minutes until cooked, then add
a **squeeze of lemon** and **season**. Serve over
the fish.

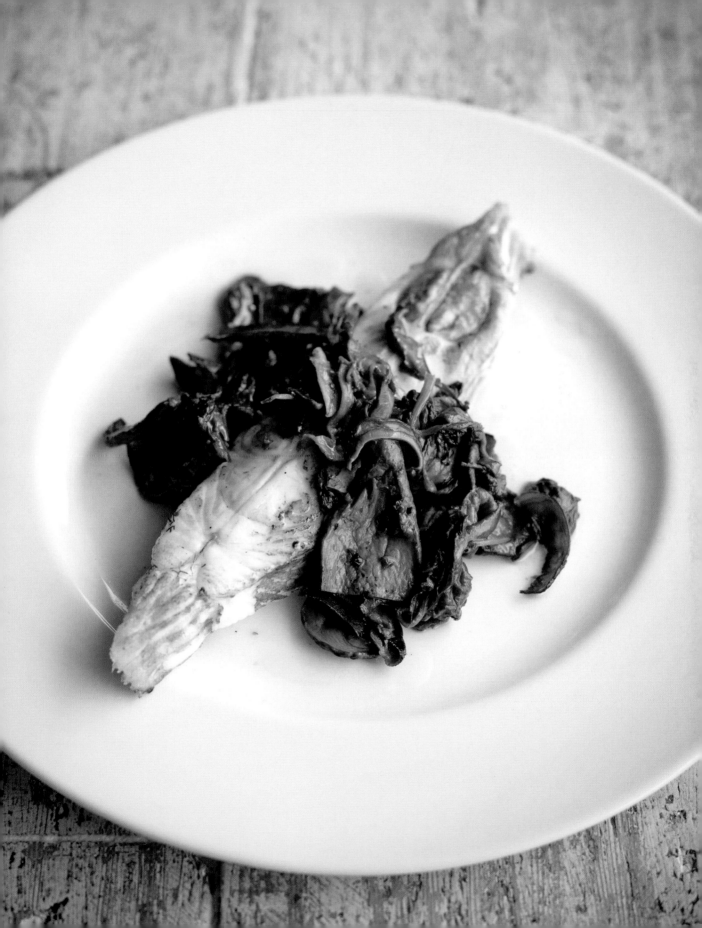

Dover sole, or its excellent relation the sand sole, is best for this dish. The quality of the fish lies in its firm gelatinous flesh. Mussels or, if you like, clams make an excellent sauce, as their juices are almost pure sea water.

sole with mussels

SERVES 2

200 g/7 oz mussels

2 tbsp plain (all-purpose) flour

2 sole, each 375–450 g/13 oz–1 lb, gutted and skinned

2 tbsp vegetable oil

15 g/½ oz/1 tbsp butter

1 garlic clove, finely chopped

1 shallot, finely chopped

1 bay leaf

splash of dry white wine

25 g/1 oz fresh herbs, such as chervil, basil, parsley and chives, finely chopped

Preheat the oven to 240°C/475°F/gas mark 9. Scrub the mussels and remove the wispy beards. Discard any shells that are broken or that are open and do not close when tapped sharply.

Lightly flour the sole on both sides. Heat a frying pan big enough to take one fish, then add 1 tbsp vegetable oil. When this is hot, fry the fish, fat side down, for 3–4 minutes until golden, then remove and place in a roasting pan. Do the same with the other fish. Transfer to the oven to cook for 6–8 minutes.

To make the sauce, melt the butter in a pan with the remaining vegetable oil, then gently sweat the garlic and shallots. Add the mussels, bay and wine, cover the pan and cook for 5 minutes, until all the shells have opened – discard any mussels that remain closed. Stir in the herbs. You can, if you wish, remove the mussels from their shells and then add them back to the sauce.

Remove the fish from the oven and place it on a serving dish, then spoon the sauce over it.

AT THE FISHMONGER
Ask your fishmonger to gut and skin
2 x 375–450 g/13 oz–1 lb sole.

Salt pastry is usually used for meat dishes, while fish is simply covered in wet salt before baking. However, after roasting a few chickens in salt pastry I tried it with fish and new-season garlic – it was delicious. The pastry is easily removed and it makes a great showpiece for fine fish.

fish in salt pastry with lemon, garlic and rosemary

SERVES 4

For the pastry
1 kg/2 lb 4 oz plain (all-purpose) flour, plus extra for dusting

600 g/1 lb 5oz rock salt

5 medium egg whites

For the fish
1 x 1.5–1.8 kg/3 lb 5 oz–4 lb wild gilt-head bream, sea bass or turbot, scaled and gutted

4 sprigs of rosemary

2 heads of new-season garlic, cut into slices from top to bottom

1 lemon, sliced

To make the pastry, mix the flour and salt in a bowl. Beat in the egg whites and enough water to make a stiff but pliable dough. Knead for 8–10 minutes, then wrap and place in the fridge to rest for 20 minutes.

Preheat the oven to 240°C/475°F/gas mark 9.

Lay the fish on a baking sheet and place the rosemary, garlic and lemon slices on top. Roll out the pastry on a lightly floured surface and place over the fish, making sure it is neatly tucked around the fish to keep the shape. You can decorate the pastry by lightly marking an eye and scales on it if you wish.

Bake for 20 minutes, then remove and leave to rest for 10 minutes. Bring to the table whole and break open the crust – the flavour and smells are wonderful. Discard the pastry; it is not for eating.

AT THE FISHMONGER
Ask your fishmonger to scale and gut 1 x 1.5–1.8 kg/ 3 lb 5 oz–4 lb gilt-head bream, sea bass or turbot.

in the oven

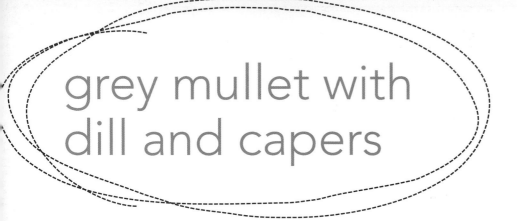

grey mullet with dill and capers

SERVES 2

This makes a nice supper with a fresh Greek salad.
Preheat the oven to 220°C/425°F/gas mark 7.
In a bowl, combine 1 finely chopped garlic clove,
a handful of fresh breadcrumbs and 1 tbsp each
of finely chopped fresh dill and capers. Stir in a
little brandy or white wine. Push this stuffing into
the belly of 1 x 450 g/1 lb scaled and gutted grey
mullet (or sea bass). Put into a roasting pan,
scatter with sea salt and drizzle with olive oil.
Roast for 15 minutes, or until cooked through.

AT THE FISHMONGER
Ask your fishmonger to scale and gut a
450 g/1 lb grey mullet (or sea bass).

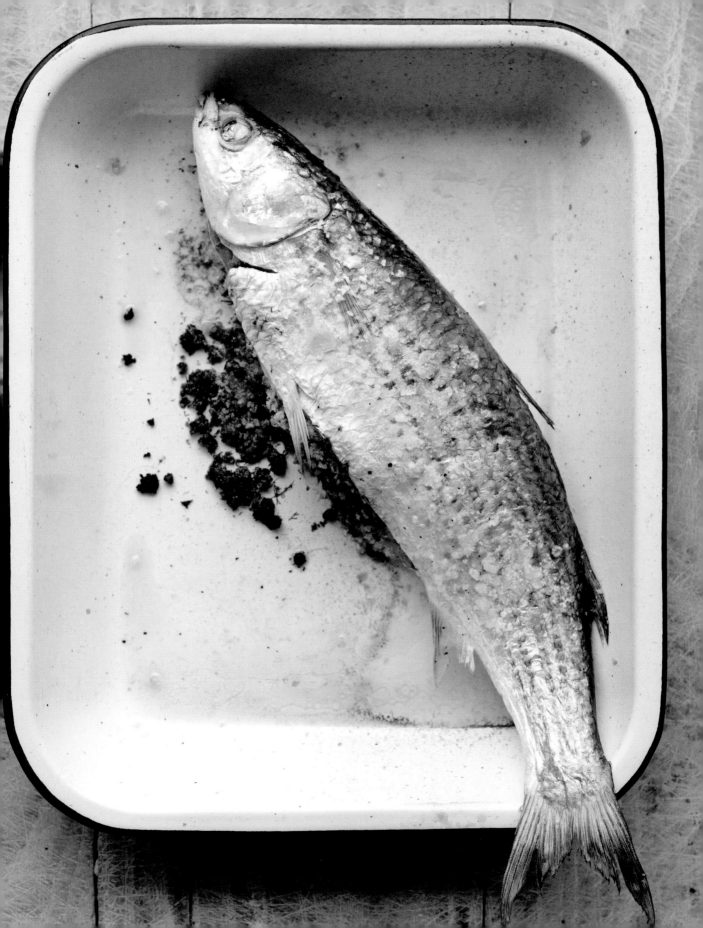

This is a popular way of roasting a whole fish in Italy and Spain, and each country has its variations. The potatoes are as important as the fish, and good waxy varieties are best. You can add onions, porcini and sliced artichoke hearts in a layer on top of the potatoes.

roast sea bass with potatoes and olives

SERVES 4

100 ml/3½ fl oz/½ cup good olive oil, plus extra for oiling

juice of 1 orange

juice of 1 lemon

sea salt and freshly ground black pepper

1 tbsp dried oregano

1 x 1.25 kg/2 lb 12 oz sea bass, scaled and gutted

200–300 g/7–10½ oz waxy potatoes, peeled and thinly sliced

4 dried bay leaves

15 black olives

150 ml/5 fl oz/⅔ cup dry white wine or light chicken stock

handful of fresh flat-leaf parsley, finely chopped

lemon wedges to serve

Mix the olive oil with the orange and lemon juice, some salt and pepper and the oregano in a bowl. Rub this mixture on to the fish, inside and out, then cover with clingfilm (plastic wrap) and marinate in the fridge for 1 hour.

Preheat the oven to 240°C/475°F/gas mark 9.

Oil a roasting pan large enough to take the fish, then lay the potato slices in it, making a layer of 10–20 cm/4–8 inch. Lay the fish on top, then pour in any remaining marinade, crumble the bay leaves over and roast for 20 minutes.

Press the olives into the potatoes, add the wine or stock and return to the oven for a further 8 minutes, or until the fish is cooked and the potatoes are crisp. Serve with a sprinkling of parsley, and lemon wedges.

AT THE FISHMONGER
Ask your fishmonger to scale and gut 1 x 1.25 kg/ 2 lb 12 oz sea bass.

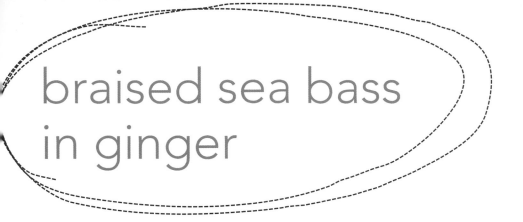

braised sea bass in ginger

SERVES 2

Very, very easy to do. Preheat the oven to 220°C/425°F/gas mark 7. In a roasting pan, make a braising liquid with 2 tbsp grated ginger, 2 tbsp grated garlic, 2 finely shredded spring onions (scallions), 200 ml/7 fl oz/scant 1 cup Tsuyu base (this is Japanese soup stock base and can be bought in most Asian supermarkets; it is quite salty so use to your taste) and 200 ml/7 fl oz/scant 1 cup fish stock or water. Simmer over a low heat for a few minutes, then add 1 x 450 g/1 lb scaled and gutted sea bass. Cover the pan with foil and transfer to the oven. Roast for 15 minutes, or until cooked. Garnish with torn coriander (cilantro) and more shredded spring onions (scallions). Serve the fish and the broth separately.

Hake is soft, white and still relatively cheap. It is a huge favourite in Spain. If you find it hard to get hold of, then pollack, cod, whiting, gurnard or sole will work well too. This is a simple combination of ingredients that makes a fine meal.

roast hake with parsley vinaigrette, aioli and boiled potatoes

SERVES 4

4 x 175 g/6 oz hake steaks, cut from the middle of the fish

2 tbsp good olive oil

plain (all-purpose) flour, for dusting

pinch of paprika

good waxy potatoes, freshly boiled, to serve

1 quantity aioli (see page 196), to serve

For the parsley vinaigrette

1 tbsp capers

pinch of mustard powder

1 tbsp white wine vinegar

squeeze of lemon juice

small handful of curly parsley, finely chopped

Preheat the oven to 230°C/450°F/gas mark 8. Turn each steak on its back and feel the 'T'-shaped bone facing upwards. Use a sharp knife to remove it from each steak; you will be left with a long fillet with 2 nice loin pieces.

Heat the olive oil in an ovenproof pan over a high heat. Lightly flour the hake and cook, flesh side down, for 2–3 minutes until golden. Turn the fish over and roast in the oven for 5 minutes, then leave to rest.

Meanwhile, whisk all the vinaigrette ingredients together. Place the fish on 4 plates and sprinkle very lightly with paprika. Pour the vinaigrette into the pan the fish was cooked in and stir around to collect all the bits and juices, then spoon over the fish.

Serve with hot, freshly boiled potatoes and a spoonful of aioli. For a variation, you can steep a pinch of saffron strands in a little warm water and stir into the aioli.

Pollack is a great fish. It's good grilled with just a little butter and perfect for fish pies. The best eating fish are the larger ones, which have lovely thick white flakes. Ask your fishmonger for the top end of the fillet.

pollack with sage, anchovy and greens

SERVES 2

2–3 tbsp vegetable oil

sea salt and freshly ground black pepper

2 pollack fillets or pieces of a large fillet, each about 175–200 g/6–7 oz

150 g/5 oz purple sprouting broccoli, kale, sprout tops or spring greens

85 g/3 oz/6 tbsp salted butter

10 fresh sage leaves

2 salted anchovy fillets

squeeze of lemon

Preheat the oven to 240°C/475°F/gas mark 9. Heat the vegetable oil in an ovenproof frying pan over a medium-high heat. Season the pollack, then fry, flesh side down, for 3–4 minutes, until golden. Turn the fish over and place the pan in the oven for 6 minutes.

Meanwhile, bring a pan of lightly salted water to the boil and cook the greens until al dente (nothing worse than soggy greens) – about 5–6 minutes.

While they are cooking, melt the butter in a separate pan over a low-medium heat, add the sage and anchovies and stir until the anchovies have melted.

Drain the greens, then toss in the anchovy butter and place on 2 plates. Remove the fish from the oven and serve the fish next to the greens. Add the lemon juice to the remaining anchovy butter in the pan and spoon over the fish.

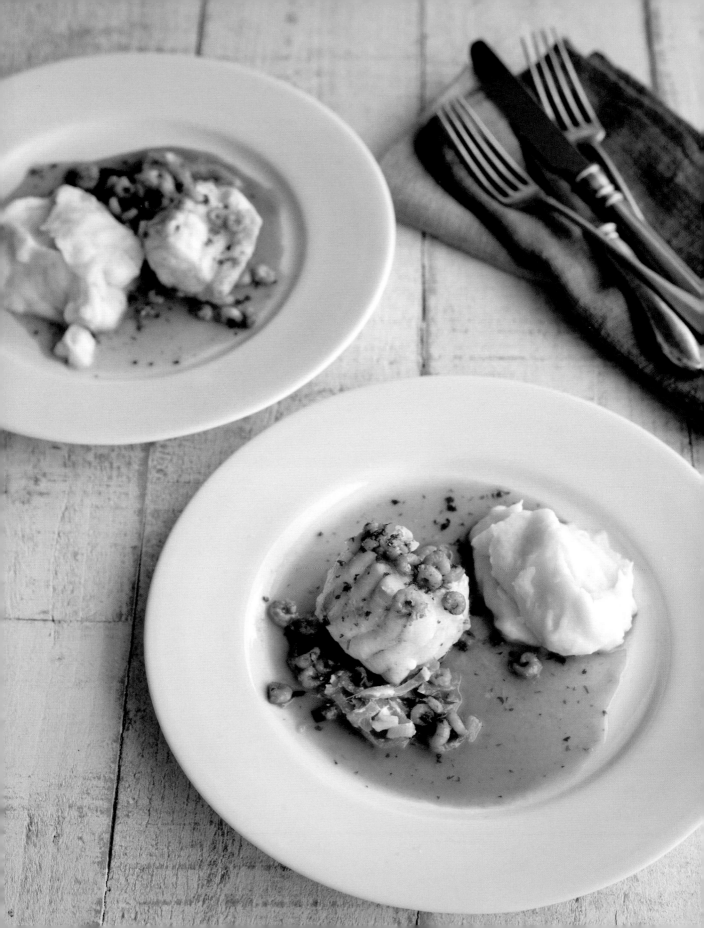

Monkfish is best cooked at hot temperatures. It has a high moisture content, so can be hard to colour when pan-frying. It works exceptionally well braised in the oven with plenty of liquid. If you find brown shrimps (small prawns) difficult to come by, then peel a few prawns (shrimp) instead.

monkfish steaks with celeriac and brown shrimps

SERVES 2

1 tbsp good olive oil

1 onion, thinly sliced

1 garlic clove, finely chopped

sprig of fresh thyme

1 bay leaf

75 ml/2½ oz/5 tbsp dry white wine

2 x 175 g/6 oz monkfish steaks, cut across the tail through the bone, leaving the bone in, skin and membrane removed

sea salt and white pepper

50 g/2 oz/¼ cup butter

pinch of mace

50 g/2 oz peeled cooked brown shrimps (small prawns)

1 tsp finely chopped fresh flat-leaf parsley

For the celeriac
400 g/14 oz floury potatoes, peeled and cut into 2.5 cm/1 in dice

400 g/14 oz celeriac (celery root), peeled and cut into 2.5 cm/1 in dice

100 g/3½ oz/½ cup butter

splash of double (heavy) cream

Preheat the oven to 200°C/400°F/gas mark 6. Heat the olive oil in an ovenproof pan. Sweat the onion and garlic with the thyme and bay leaf over a low heat until soft. Add the wine, increase the heat to high and boil off the alcohol – this should take 2 minutes. Place the fish on top of the onion, season with sea salt and white pepper and cover, then roast for 20 minutes.

Meanwhile, for the celariac, put the potatoes and celeriac in a saucepan with plenty of salted boiling water. Boil for about 10 minutes, or until soft. Drain and mix with the butter and cream, then mash and season.

Place the fish on 2 or 4 plates with a good spoonful of the celariac. Heat the butter in a pan until it is foaming, add the mace, shrimps and parsley and spoon over the fish.

AT THE FISHMONGER
Ask your fishmonger to remove the skin and membrane from
2 x 175 g/6 oz monkfish tails.

This is a nice way of cooking a whole monkfish tail. I am using a lot of sage at the moment because I have it growing everywhere, and I really like it with meaty fish. However, you could substitute tarragon, parsley or even basil.

monkfish with sage and roasted garlic

SERVES 4

30 garlic cloves

olive oil

a sprig of rosemary

sea salt and freshly ground black pepper

1 x 1 kg/2 lb 4 oz monkfish tail on the bone, skin and membrane removed

200 ml/7 fl oz/scant 1 cup water, vegetable or chicken stock

8 sage leaves

100 ml/3½ fl oz/½ cup double (heavy) cream

Preheat the oven to 220°C/425°F/gas mark 7. Put the garlic cloves in a piece of foil with a drizzle of olive oil and the sprig of rosemary and fold the edges of the foil together to seal. Place on a baking sheet and roast for 20 minutes, until the cloves are soft. Leave until cool enough to handle then squeeze half the cloves out of their papery skins and mash to a purée; put the rest to one side.

Increase the oven to 240°C/475°F/gas mark 9. Put a frying pan over a high heat and add 2 tbsp olive oil. Season the fish, then brown it in the oil on all sides for 3–4 minutes in total, until coloured. Transfer to a roasting pan and roast for 15 minutes.

Meanwhile, put the garlic purée, whole garlic cloves, water or stock, sage leaves and cream into a pan and whisk together, then simmer for 5 minutes and season to taste.

Pour the sauce over the fish and return it to the oven for a further 5–8 minutes, basting regularly with the sauce, until the fish is cooked through. The sauce should reduce and become very flavoursome as it mixes with the roasting juices from the fish.

AT THE FISHMONGER
Ask your fishmonger to remove the skin and membrane from 1 x 1 kg/2 lb 4 oz monkfish tail.

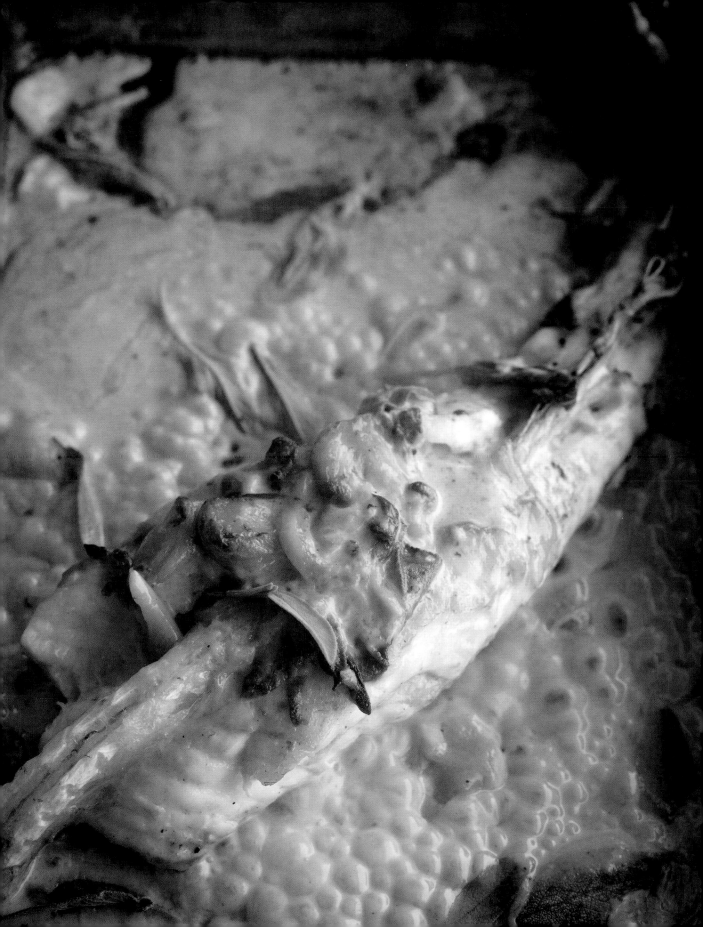

This recipe is as much about the celery as the gurnard. This is a very good light stew-style dish.

gurnard with braised celery and cider

SERVES 4

50 g/2 oz/4 tbsp butter
1 onion, thinly sliced
4 celery sticks (stalks), halved, and lots of leaves, roughly chopped
a sprig of thyme
2 tbsp plain (all-purpose) flour
200 ml/7 fl oz/scant 1 cup dry cider
100 ml/3½ fl oz/½ cup vegetable or chicken stock
1 large gurnard, filleted and pinboned
sea salt and freshly ground black pepper
handful of fresh flat-leaf parsley, finely chopped

Preheat the oven to 180°C/350°F/gas mark 4.

Heat the butter in an ovenproof pan over a low heat, then add the onion and cook for 8 minutes until softened. Add the celery sticks and thyme and cook for 3–4 minutes. Stir in the flour and cook for 2 minutes, then gradually add the cider and stock, stirring all the time. Increase the heat to medium and cook, stirring, for another 2–3 minutes, or until the sauce thickens. Cover and transfer to the oven for 25 minutes, until the celery is soft and tender.

Cut the gurnard into large chunks or leave small fillets whole, then add them to the pan. Cover and bake for a further 10 minutes. Season with salt and freshly ground black pepper to taste, stir in plenty of chopped parsley and celery leaves and serve.

AT THE FISHMONGER
Ask your fishmonger for a 'tub' gurnard – these are the bigger ones and are particularly good to eat. Ask him to fillet and pinbone it for you.

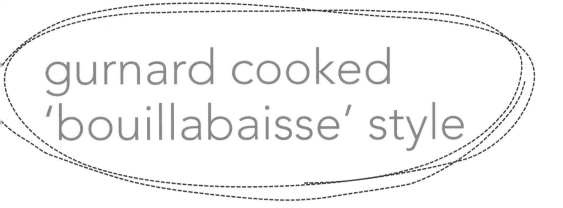

gurnard cooked 'bouillabaisse' style

SERVES 4

Begin by making the red mullet soup on page 74. Preheat the oven to 150°C/300°F/gas mark 2. Pull off and discard the tough outer layers of **1 fennel bulb**, then cut it into 6 wedges through the root. Parboil in lightly salted water for 8–10 minutes, then drain. Parboil **100 g/3½ oz waxy potatoes** for 10 minutes, then drain. Put **3–4 small scaled, gutted and deheaded gurnard** into a casserole with the potatoes and fennel. Sprinkle with **finely chopped fresh parsley**. Ladle in enough of the soup to nearly cover the fish, adding a little water if your soup is thick, then cover and bake for 35–40 minutes. Serve the fish with **aioli** and **lemon wedges**, then enjoy the broth spooned over grilled **bread** rubbed with **garlic** and **olive oil**.

'Agrodolce' is the Italian word for 'bitter–sweet'. At my restaurant The Seahorse we use very good vinegars that have sweetness in them, and at least 12-year-old balsamic vinegar. If you find it hard to get very high-quality vinegars, dissolve a little sugar in white wine vinegar until the sharp edge has gone. The sweetness of the lightly caramelized onion with the salty capers adds a nice dimension to this dish.

gurnard with onions and capers in agrodolce

SERVES 2

50 g/2 oz/4 tbsp salted butter

1 onion, thinly sliced

1 tbsp olive oil

sea salt and freshly ground black pepper

2 small gurnard, skinned, gutted and deheaded

5 tbsp white wine vinegar (sweet or sweetened)

2 tbsp balsamic vinegar

small handful of salted capers, rinsed

1 tbsp finely chopped fresh flat-leaf parsley

Preheat the oven to 240°C/475°F/gas mark 9.

Melt the butter in a saucepan and cook the onion gently for 8 minutes.

Meanwhile, heat the olive oil in an ovenproof pan and place over a high heat. Season the fish and cook in the oil, flesh side down, for 3–4 minutes, until browned. Transfer to the oven and bake for a further 8 minutes, until cooked through.

Turn the heat under the onions to high and wait until it foams then dies down – about a minute. Add your sweetened vinegar – it will really sizzle. Next, add the balsamic vinegar, then the capers and parsley and cook for 30 seconds. Pour over the fish as you serve it.

AT THE FISHMONGER
Ask your fishmonger to skin, gut and dehead 2 small gurnard.

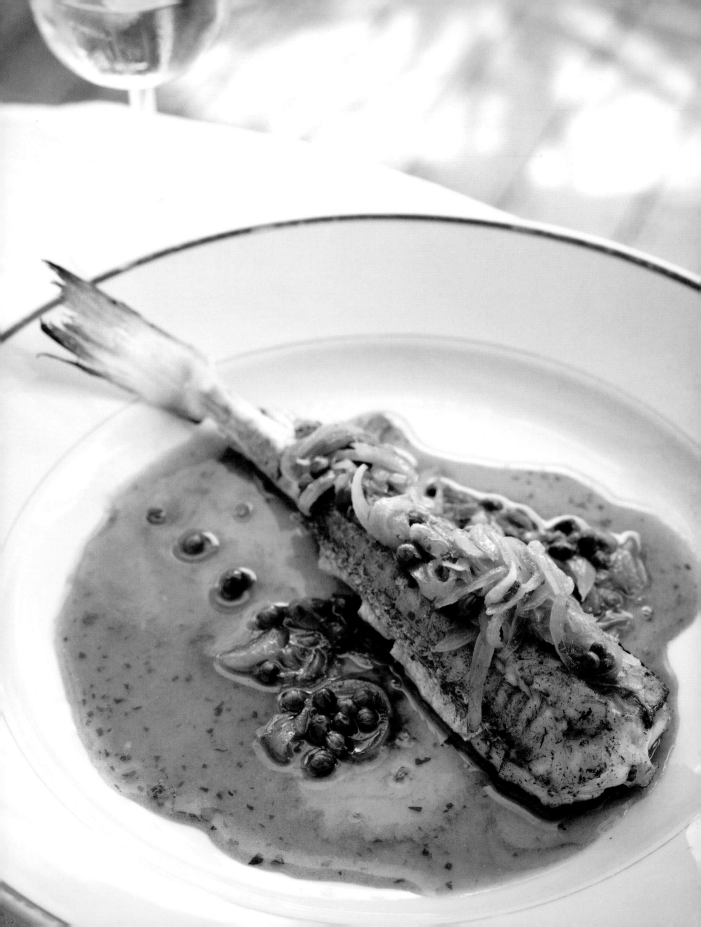

In Sicily it is typical for Marsala wine to be used in cooking seafood, especially prawns (shrimp). I think the sweetness of both means they work well together.

gurnard with roasted prawns and Marsala

SERVES 4

1 tbsp olive oil

4 x 150 g/5½ oz gurnard fillets, pinboned and skinned

25 g/1 oz/2 tbsp butter

2 garlic cloves, finely chopped

16–20 raw prawns (shrimp), peeled with the tail left on, and deveined

50 ml/2 fl oz/4 tbsp Marsala wine

1 tbsp double (heavy) cream

small handful of fresh flat-leaf parsley, finely chopped

sea salt and freshly ground black pepper

Preheat the oven to 220°C/425°F/gas mark 7. Heat the oil in an ovenproof pan over a high heat, then fry the gurnard fillets until browned – 3–4 minutes. Add the butter and, when it has melted, add the garlic and then the prawns. Transfer to the oven and roast for 5–6 minutes, until the prawns are pink and cooked.

Remove from the oven, add the Marsala and quickly boil off the alcohol over a high heat. Remove from the heat, stir in the cream and parsley, season and serve.

AT THE FISHMONGER
Ask your fishmonger to skin and pinbone the gurnard fillets.

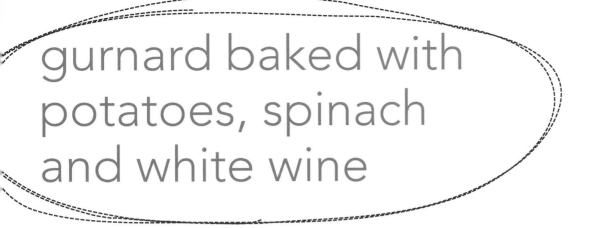

gurnard baked with potatoes, spinach and white wine

SERVES 2

Preheat the oven to 240°C/475°F/gas mark 9. Take a roasting pan large enough to hold the fish and lightly smear it with olive oil. Peel and slice **2 large potatoes** about 1 cm/½ in thick. Place half in a layer in the bottom of the tin. Thinly slice **2 garlic cloves**. Sprinkle the garlic over the potatoes, then lay **50 g/2 oz cooked spinach** over the garlic. Place the remaining potato on top, then lay **2 x 200 g/ 7 oz gurnard fillets** on the potatoes, flesh side down, and season. Pour over **100 ml/3½ fl oz/ ½ cup olive oil**. Roast for 6 minutes, then add **125 ml/4 fl oz/½ cup dry white wine**. Roast for a further 5–6 minutes, until the potatoes are crisp and the wine absorbed.

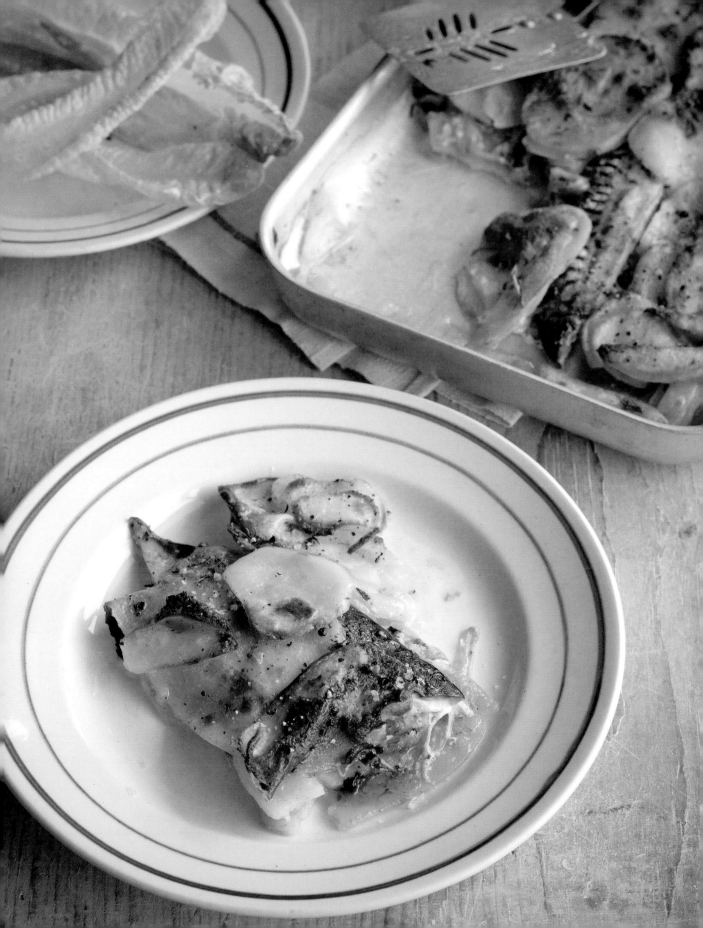

This is a nice way to treat fresh mackerel and makes a homely supper.

baked mackerel with potatoes and thyme

SERVES 4

50 g/2 oz/4 tbsp butter, plus a little
extra for topping the potatoes

olive oil

2 onions, thinly sliced

4 salted anchovy fillets

4 potatoes, thinly sliced

8 mackerel fillets, pinboned

1 tbsp fresh thyme leaves

freshly ground black pepper

dressed green leaves to serve

Preheat the oven to 220°C/425°F/gas mark 7. Melt half the butter with a little olive oil in a pan over a low heat and fry the onions until soft and golden – about 8 minutes. Add the anchovies and cook until they have dissolved, then remove the onions and anchovies and set aside. Add a little more oil and the remaining butter to the pan and cook the potatoes in the same way until crisp on the edges and just cooked – about 6 minutes.

Place half the potatoes in a layer in a roasting pan, then lay the fish fillets on top and sprinkle with thyme and pepper. Lay the onion and anchovy mix on top, then finish with the remaining potatoes. Add about 150 ml/5 fl oz/⅔ cup water, then dot with butter and bake for 10–12 minutes, until the mackerel is cooked and the potatoes are crisp.

Serve with green leaves dressed with a light vinaigrette.

AT THE FISHMONGER
Ask your fishmonger to pinbone 8 mackerel fillets.

Squid (calamari) are delicious stuffed. You can use a multitude of flavours, with breadcrumbs and herbs as the base. The braising liquid can be anything from white wine and olive oil to a tomato base perhaps with fennel and oregano.

roast squid stuffed with mussels, lemon and spinach

SERVES 4

500 g/1 lb 2 oz mussels

450 g/1 lb fresh spinach

2 garlic cloves, finely chopped

olive oil

75 ml/2½ fl oz/5 tbsp dry white wine

1 dried chilli (chile)

handful of fresh white breadcrumbs

juice of 1 lemon

sea salt and freshly ground black pepper

pinch of freshly grated nutmeg

2 tbsp chopped fresh flat-leaf parsley

8 medium squid (calamari), with tentacles cut off and reserved, cleaned and skinned

garlic, lemon and parsley dressing (see page 51), to serve

green salad to serve

Preheat the oven to 240°C/475°F/gas mark 9. Scrub the mussels and remove the wispy beards. Discard any shells that are broken or that are open and do not close when tapped sharply.

Put the mussels in a large pan with a little water, cover and steam for 3–4 minutes, until they open. Remove them from the shells. Discard any that remain closed. Strain the liquid to remove any grit, and reserve.

Wash the spinach and cook it over a low-medium heat in the water still clinging to it for 2–3 minutes. Drain and finely chop. Fry the garlic in 1 tbsp olive oil over a medium heat for 2–3 minutes, or until it starts to brown. Add the spinach and wine and boil for 2 minutes to cook off the alcohol. Take off the heat.

Crumble in the chilli, then add the breadcrumbs and mussels and moisten with the reserved mussel liquid and the lemon juice to make a workable stuffing. Season and add the nutmeg and parsley, then stuff the squid with the mixture, securing the ends with a cocktail stick if you wish.

Heat 1 tbsp olive oil in an ovenproof frying pan over a high heat, then sear the stuffed squid and tentacles on all sides until golden – approximately 3–4 minutes in total. Transfer to the oven and roast for 6–7 minutes, or until cooked. Drizzle with the garlic, lemon and parsley dressing and serve with a green salad.

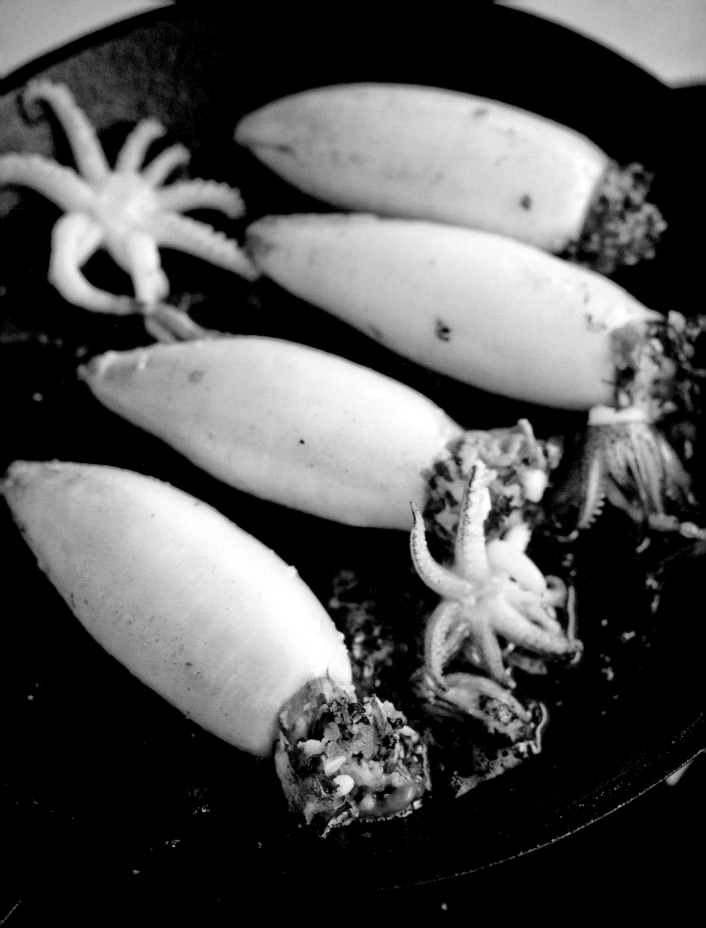

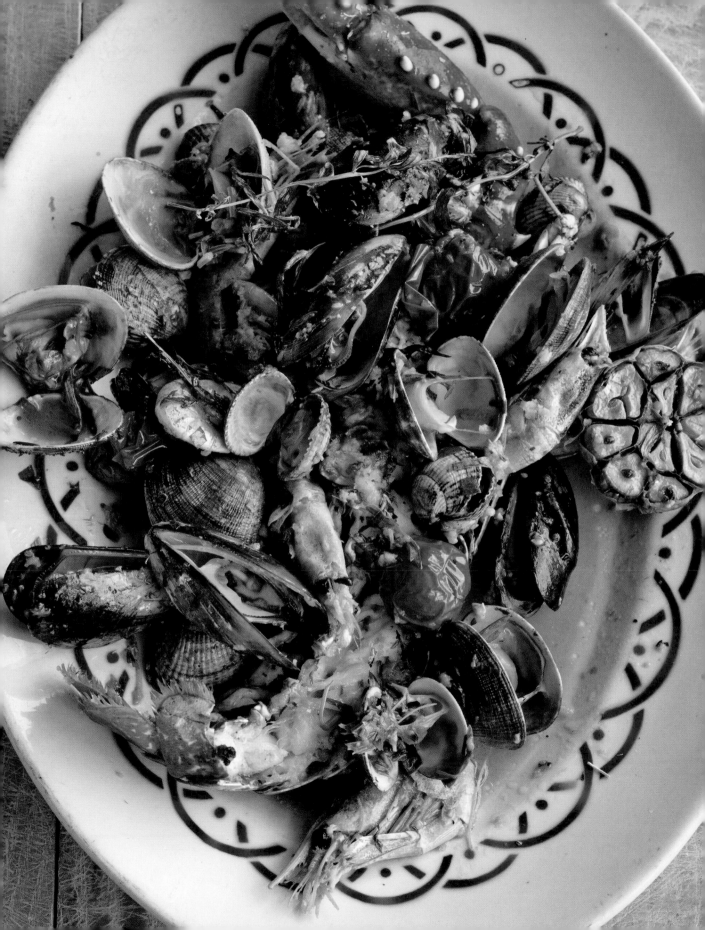

roast shellfish with tarragon and balsamic

SERVES 1

Preheat the oven to 220°C/425°F/gas mark 7. Wash a handful each of mussels, clams, prawns and cockles and remove the wispy beards from the mussels. The shells of the clams, mussels and cockles should be closed or should close if you tap them sharply; discard any that remain open or are broken. Heat 2 tbsp olive oil in a roasting pan over a medium heat, add a halved garlic bulb, flesh side down, and cook for 2–3 minutes. Add the shellfish, 8 cherry tomatoes, 1–2 tbsp balsamic vinegar and a splash of dry white wine, then roast for 10–12 minutes, until the shells are open (discard any that remain closed). Stir in chopped tarragon and a few more tbsp of balsamic vinegar, then whisk 20 g/¾ oz/2 tbsp butter into the sauce and pour over the fish.

This lobster casserole relies on the shells to give it a rich Mediterranean flavour. A crawfish would make a real treat but they are hard to come by these days. 'Caldereta' is the name of the pot the lobster is cooked in. I have an old clay one with a heavy lid and it works really well for this slow cooking – the development of the flavour while it cooks is really wonderful.

slow-cooked lobster caldereta

SERVES 2

1 live lobster or crawfish, 650 g/1 lb 7 oz

4 small ripe tomatoes

2 tbsp olive oil

1 onion, finely chopped

2 garlic cloves, crushed to a paste

1 red (bell) pepper, deseeded and finely chopped

1 tbsp brandy

1 tbsp dry white wine

1 litre/1¾ pints/4 cups shellfish stock (see page 208)

1 bay leaf

pinch of dried oregano

pinch of saffron strands

pinch of paprika

small handful of fresh flat-leaf parsley, finely chopped

sea salt

grilled bread to serve

saffron mayonnaise (see page 202) or aioli to serve (see page 196)

Place the lobster on a chopping board. Insert a large, sharp, heavy knife into the cross on the back of the head and cut down towards the tail, cutting it in half. Remove the stomach and the black intestinal tract (if there is one) that may run through the middle of the tail and discard. Remove the meat from the shell and roughly chop it.

Preheat the oven to 150°C/300°F/gas mark 2. To skin the tomatoes, pierce them with a knife, then drop them into a bowl of just-boiled water for 2 minutes. Remove from the water with a spoon, leave to cool for a few seconds, then peel off the skins and deseed and roughly chop the flesh.

Heat the olive oil in a casserole dish. Fry the lobster chunks for 3–4 minutes, then remove and set aside – this process adds flavour to the oil. Add the onion, garlic, red pepper and chopped tomatoes and fry gently for 8–10 minutes, until softened and cooked right down. Add the brandy, increase the heat and boil off the alcohol, then do the same with the wine. Add the stock, lobster, bay leaf, oregano, saffron and paprika and bring to the boil. Cover and cook in the oven for 2 hours.

Sprinkle with parsley and salt and serve with grilled bread and saffron mayonnaise or aioli.

salt cod and onions

SERVES 4

Preheat the oven to 220°C/425°F/gas mark 7. Prepare 600 g/1 lb 5 oz salt cod (see pages 162–5). Cut it into 4 portions and dry well, then dip in plain (all-purpose) flour and fry in a little olive oil over a medium heat for 5–6 minutes, until golden. Transfer to a roasting pan and roast for 8–10 minutes, until cooked. Meanwhile, heat 1 tbsp olive oil in a pan over a low heat, then sauté 1 finely chopped onion with 1 bay leaf until starting to turn golden brown. Add 1 finely chopped garlic clove and cook for a further 5–10 minutes. Add a good splash of white wine vinegar and allow it to reduce for 2 minutes, then stir in 1 tbsp finely chopped fresh flat-leaf parsley. Serve the onions with the salt cod.

roasted scallops with thyme and coral butter

SERVES 2 TO START

Preheat the oven to 230°C/450°F/gas mark 8. Remove the roes from **6 scallops** in the cup shell and take off the white muscle and any black bits. Place the roes in a food processor with **150 g/ 5½ oz/¾ cup softened butter** and **1 finely chopped garlic clove**. Blitz together, then stir in **1 tbsp fresh thyme leaves**. Place a spoonful on each scallop, add **1 tbsp dry white wine**, then sprinkle **a thin layer of fine fresh breadcrumbs** over each shell and bake for 6 minutes, until crisp and golden. Season with **sea salt**.

AT THE FISHMONGER
Ask the fishmonger to open the scallops on the cup side of the shells rather than on the flat side. If they have already been opened on the flat side, ask for 6 cup shells, so that you can transfer the scallop meat to them.

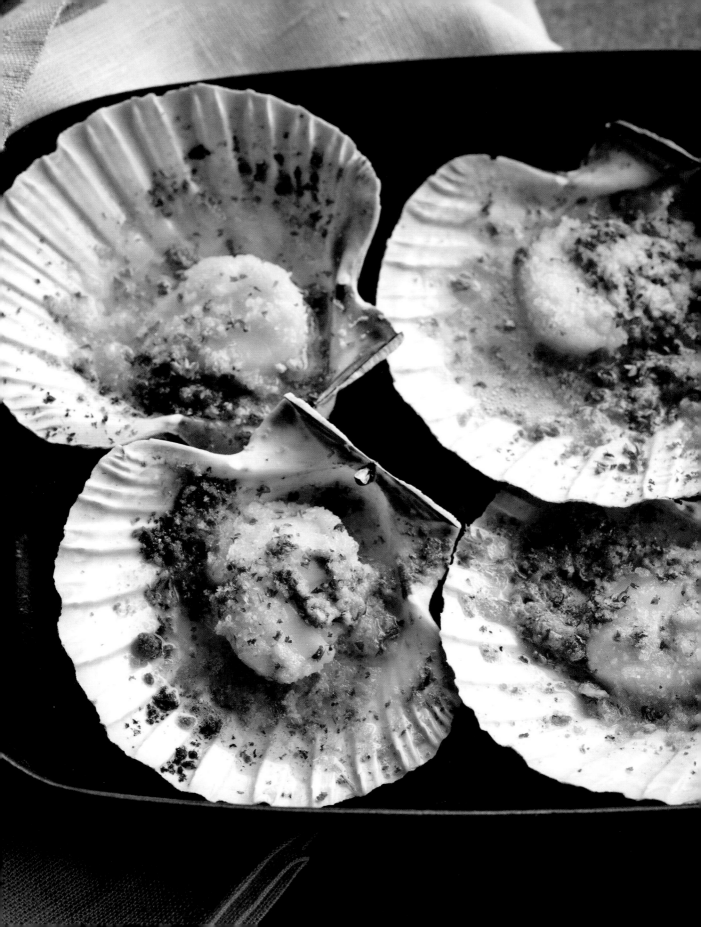

I love the baked rice dishes of Spain. This one uses just crab and tastes delicious. It is best made with shellfish stock but this can be time consuming so a good vegetable or chicken stock can be used instead.

baked rice with crab and sherry

SERVES 4

Shellfish stock
2 kg/4 lb 8 oz crab or lobster shells

2 carrots, roughly chopped

1 fennel bulb, roughly chopped

2 celery sticks (stalks), roughly chopped

1 tbsp olive oil

1 tbsp fennel seeds

4 tbsp tomato purée

2 bay leaves

For the rice
2 cooked crabs

2 tbsp olive oil

½ onion, finely chopped

1 red pepper, deseeded and finely chopped

2 garlic cloves, finely chopped

pinch of paprika

3 tomatoes, roughly chopped

good pinch of saffron strands

splash of dry sherry

300 g /10½ oz paella rice

2 tbsp finely chopped fresh curly parsley

800 ml/1½ pints/4 cups shellfish stock or good vegetable or chicken stock

Preheat the oven to 220°C/425°F/gas mark 7. For the stock, put the shells in a roasting pan and roast for 30 minutes; the kitchen will smell nicely of shellfish. Turn the oven off.

Meanwhile, cook the vegetables in a large saucepan or stockpot in the olive oil over a medium-high heat until they are just lightly browned and golden. Stir in the fennel seeds and cook for 1 minute. Add the tomato purée and bay leaves and cook for a further 2–3 minutes. Add the shells, cover with approximately 3 litres/5¼ pints/5 quarts water and simmer very gently, lid on, for 2–3 hours. Strain, then boil to reduce by half.

Preheat the oven to 160°C/325°F/gas mark 3. Now tackle your crabs. Prise them open, pick out the brown meat and set it aside. Discard the top shell, remove the 'dead men's fingers' (the crab's gills, which are attached to the exposed body), and chop the carapace (shell and meat) into quarters. Crack the claws. Heat the olive oil in a large ovenproof frying pan. Add the onion, red (bell) pepper and garlic and fry until really soft. Add the paprika, tomatoes and saffron, stir, then add the sherry. Cook for 3–4 minutes, then sprinkle the rice into the pan and stir in the brown crab meat. Place the pieces of crab in the rice, add the stock and simmer for 2 minutes. Transfer to the oven and cook for 15 minutes, or until all the stock has been absorbed.

Scatter with the parsley, then cover with wet greaseproof (wax) paper and let it stand for 10 minutes before serving.

I love razor clams, and we get some fantastic ones around the British shores. For braises like this I like to use the largest ones I can get.

braised razor clams with parsley, sherry and peas

SERVES 4

2 tbsp olive oil

2 onions, thinly sliced

1 garlic clove, finely chopped

2 slices of prosciutto or unsmoked pancetta, cut into small matchsticks

200 ml/7 fl oz good light chicken stock

200 ml/7 fl oz fino or manzanilla sherry

handful of frozen or fresh peas

8 large razor clams, well washed

white pepper

handful of coriander (cilantro) leaves, roughly chopped

4 slices of fried bread

Preheat the oven to 180°C/350°F/gas mark 4. Heat the oil in a large ovenproof pan over a low heat. Add the onions and garlic and sweat for 8–10 minutes, or until soft and golden. Add the prosciutto and stir. Add the stock, sherry and peas and simmer for 4–5 minutes.

Lay the razor clams on top in a single layer (diacard any that are open and that don't close when handled), cover and transfer to the oven for 8 10 minutes. Season with white pepper. Serve sprinkled with the coriander, with the fried bread on the bottom. (Discard any clams that fail to open when cooked).

cooking in a bag

'Cooking in a bag' does not sound as appetizing as the French 'en papillotte' or Italian 'al cartoccio', but the method is the same. Cooking this way keeps the fish moist and whatever you cook in the bag with it will make a delicious sauce or accompaniment. Pasta, for example, part-cooked then finished in a bag with shellfish, is very good. Use foil and baking parchment: this will make a strong bag and will also help create a good seal.

Cut a square of foil and a square of baking parchment, slightly larger than you need to hold the fish and ingredients. Lay the parchment on top of the foil, then lay the fish and everything else in the middle of it. Fold up the sides, add any oils, butter (I like to use homemade flavoured butters) or liquid, then, starting at one corner, crimp the edges of the bag together to make a half moon shape. Fold the edges together to seal. Place in a roasting pan and cook according to the recipe. Just before serving, open the parcel and spoon the sauce over the fish, then finish with a sprinkling of fresh herbs. You can cook a piece of fish from frozen in this way – just remember that it will release more liquid than when unfrozen.

Brill is a good firm fish (not as firm as turbot but a very good substitute in any recipe that calls for it). Wine with body and a little sweetness is particularly good with fish. I like the Italian word for cooking fish in a paper parcel – 'al cartoccio' – sounds nicer than 'in paper'.

brill cooked 'al cartoccio' with leeks and Riesling

SERVES 2

25 g/1 oz/2 tbsp butter

1 celery stick (stalk), peeled and finely sliced

a few fresh tarragon leaves

a few spring onions (scallions), finely sliced

2 young leeks, cut into fine julienne

100 ml/3½ fl oz/½ cup Riesling or similar aromatic dry white wine

2 x 280 g/10 oz brill fillets or steaks (or halibut, sole or flounder)

2 sprigs of thyme

sea salt and freshly ground black pepper

Preheat the oven to 240°C/475°F/gas mark 9. Heat the butter in a saucepan over a low heat, then gently cook the celery, tarragon, spring onions and leeks for 6–8 minutes, until softened.

Cut 2 pieces of parchment paper and 2 pieces of foil big enough to wrap 1 fish fillet. Place a piece of parchment on top of each piece of foil, then place half the leek mixture in the middle of each one. Fold up the sides, add half the wine to each and place the fish on top with a sprig of thyme and some seasoning. Seal the parcels, place in a roasting pan and bake for 12 minutes, until cooked through. Open the parcels and serve.

sea bream with roasted garlic, chilli and rosemary

SERVES 2

Preheat the oven to 240°C/475°F/gas mark 9. Place a 450 g/1 lb scaled and gutted sea bream on the parchment and foil (see page 138). Add 4 roasted garlic cloves or sliced raw garlic, 2 sprigs of rosemary and 1 crumbled dried chilli (chile) or 1 chopped fresh chilli and season with salt and freshly ground black pepper. Fold up the sides and add 3 tbsp olive oil and 4 tbsp dry white wine, then seal securely. Place on a baking tray and cook for 15 minutes. Remove from the oven, open the parcels and squeeze on some lemon juice.

AT THE FISHMONGER
Ask your fishmonger to scale and gut 1 x 450 g/1 lb sea bream.

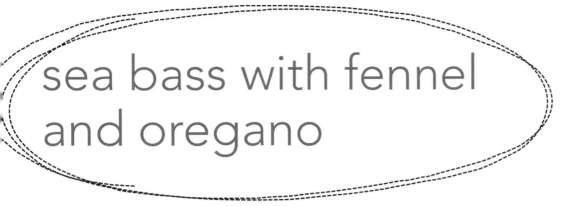

sea bass with fennel and oregano

SERVES 2

Use **1 x 450 g/1 lb sea bass**, scaled and gutted, for this (fillets will also work well, just adjust the cooking time to 8–10 minutes). Preheat the oven to 240°C/475°F/gas mark 9. Cut **1 fennel bulb** into 6 wedges and place in a pan with **100 ml/3½ fl oz/ ½ cup olive oil** and **the same amount of dry white wine**. Add **1 bay leaf** and **a few coriander seeds**. Cook for 10–20 minutes, until the fennel is soft, then allow to cool in the liquid. Lay the fennel on the parchment and foil (see page 138), then place the fish on top and sprinkle with **sea salt** and **ground fennel seeds**. Fold up the sides, then spoon the juices in which the fennel was cooked over the fish, add **a sprig or 2 of oregano** and seal securely. Place on a baking tray and cook for 15 minutes.

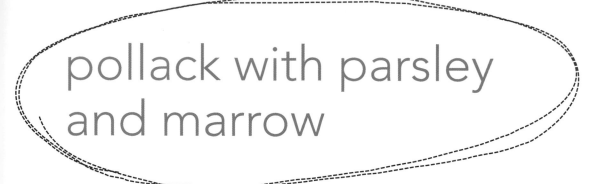

pollack with parsley and marrow

SERVES 1

Marrow is a delightful vegetable. It cooks in no time and is particularly good with butter and black pepper. Preheat the oven to 240°C/475°F/gas mark 9. Cut **200 g/7 oz marrow flesh** into 1 cm/½ in cubes. Melt **a knob of butter** in a pan and sauté the marrow with **1 tbsp very finely sliced white onion** for 5 minutes, then add **1 tbsp chopped fresh curly parsley**. Place on the parchment and foil (see page 138), put a **200 g/7 oz skinned and pinboned pollack fillet** on top, then add **a knob of butter**, grind plenty of **black pepper** over and seal securely. Place on a baking tray and cook for 8–10 minutes.

AT THE FISHMONGER
Ask your fishmonger to skin and pinbone
1 pollack fillet.

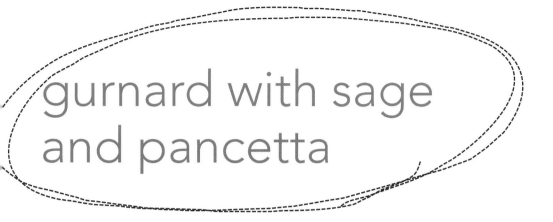

gurnard with sage and pancetta

SERVES 1

Preheat the oven to 240°C/475°F/gas mark 9. Heat 2 tbsp olive oil in a pan. Fry 6–7 baby onions with 1 chopped garlic clove, 25 g/1 oz chopped pancetta and 4 chopped sage leaves. Place on the parchment and foil (see page 138), put a 200 g/7 oz skinned and pinboned gurnard fillet on top, then add a small knob of butter or olive oil and seal securely. Place on a baking tray and cook for 10 minutes.

AT THE FISHMONGER
Ask your fishmonger to skin and pinbone
a 200 g/7 oz gurnard fillet.

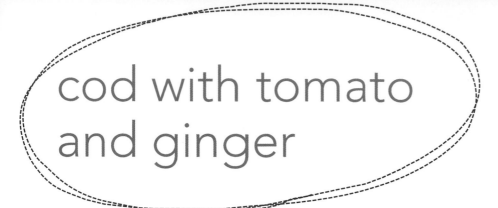

cod with tomato and ginger

SERVES 1

Preheat the oven to 240°C/475°F/gas mark 9.
Gently cook a grated thumb-sized piece of ginger,
1 grated garlic clove and 1 small finely sliced
onion in 2 tbsp olive oil until softened. Add
a pinch of ground cumin and a few grinds of
black pepper and squeeze in 4 very ripe skinned
tomatoes. Simmer for 4–5 minutes, then taste
and season. Stir in 1 tbsp lemon juice and a small
handful of chopped fresh coriander (cilantro).
Place on the parchment and foil (see page 138),
then put a 200 g/7 oz skinned and pinboned fillet
of cod on top. Fold up the sides, add a drizzle of
olive oil and seal securely. Place on a baking tray
and cook for 8–10 minutes.

AT THE FISHMONGER
Ask your fishmonger to skin and pinbone 1 cod fillet.

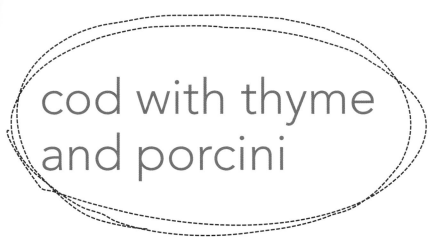

cod with thyme and porcini

SERVES 1

Preheat the oven to 240°C/475°F/gas mark 9. Soak 5–6 dried porcini in just-boiled water for 15 minutes, then squeeze out the water, drain and mix with 8–10 sliced fresh mushrooms. Toss with 2 tbsp olive oil, a few fresh thyme leaves, salt and freshly ground pepper. Place on the parchment and foil (see page 138), then put a 200 g/7 oz skinned and pinboned fillet of cod cut from the thick end on top and add a knob of butter. Fold up the sides, add a splash of sherry and seal securely. Place on a baking tray and cook for about 10 minutes.

AT THE FISHMONGER
Ask your fishmonger to skin and pinbone 1 cod fillet.

baked spaghetti and clams

SERVES 1

Pasta cooked this way is delicious, as it really soaks up all the juices. Preheat the oven to 220°C/425°F/gas mark 7. Half-cook 75 g/2½ oz spaghetti and toss with 20 clams (discard any whose shells are broken or open and fail to close when tapped sharply), 1 crumbled dried chilli (chile), 2 garlic cloves and 1 tbsp finely chopped fresh flat-leaf parsley. Place them on the parchment and foil (see page 138) and seal securely. Place on a baking tray and cook for 8–10 minutes. Open the parcels and discard any clams that remain closed. Serve with a squeeze of lemon and a sprinkling of finely chopped fresh parsley. This also works well with a few skinned tomatoes and some whole roasted garlic cloves thrown in.

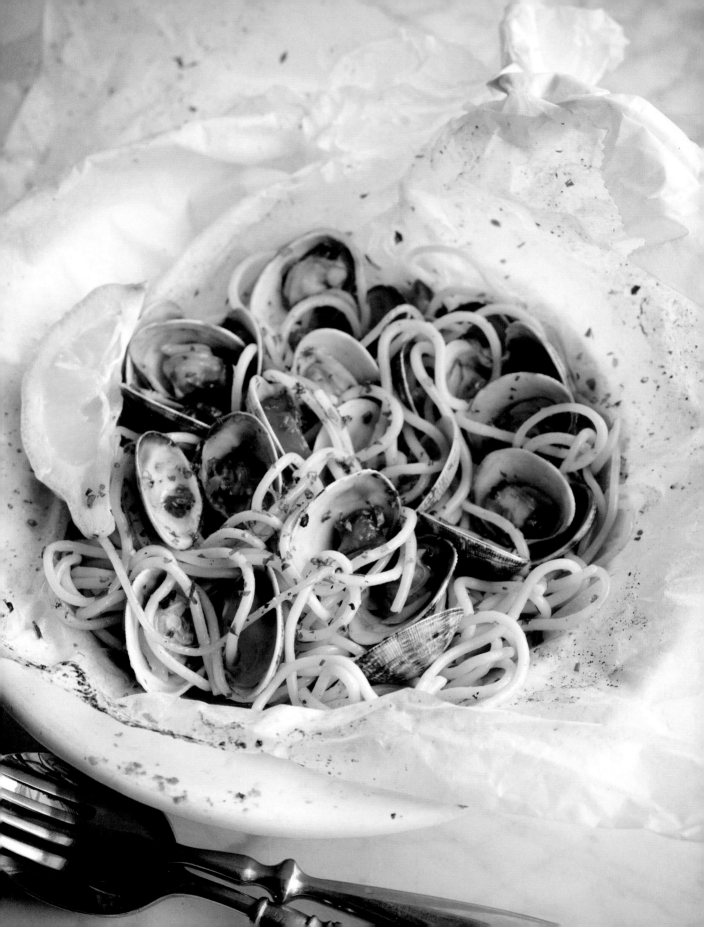

scallops and mussels

SERVES 1

Preheat the oven to 240°C/475°F/gas mark 9. Place **4 cleaned scallops** on the parchment and foil (see page 138) with **12 cleaned mussels** (discard any whose shells are broken or open and fail to close when tapped sharply), **a small handful of finely chopped fresh flat-leaf parsley, 1 finely chopped garlic clove, 2 tbsp dry white wine** and **a knob of butter.** Seal securely, place on a baking tray and cook for 7–8 minutes. Once the bag is opened, discard any mussels that remain closed. A nice bowl of aioli (see page 196) is great with this, or try adding some fennel as prepared on page 141.

New England-style clam bake

SERVES 4

Preheat the oven to 240°C/475°F/gas mark 9. Slice 2 sweetcorn into 1 cm/½ in rounds and parboil for 8 minutes. Boil 200 g/7 oz new potatoes for 10 minutes, then drain and cut into quarters. Put the potatoes, sweetcorn, 500 g/1 lb 2 oz cleaned clams, the same weight of cleaned mussels and 100 g/3½ oz sliced chorizo on the parchment and foil (see page 138). Discard any mussels and clams whose shells are broken or open and fail to close when tapped sharply. Season with celery salt and freshly ground black pepper, fold up the sides, add 4 tbsp dry white wine and seal. Place on a baking tray and cook for 10–12 minutes. Discard any shellfish that remain closed. Sprinkle with chopped fresh parsley and serve with a bowl of melted butter with lemon juice to dip the clams and veg in.

raw, cured and salads

raw and cured fish

Curing fish is easy and the results are delicious. I used to be nervous about doing it, but once I got into it I realised just how easy it was. Even a simple dousing of salt for 30 minutes, washed off before cooking, can change the flavour and texture of a piece of fish.

The basic principle is to remove moisture from the fish to prevent spoilage and inhibit the growth of bacteria. The longer you salt and dry something, the longer it will keep – traditional salt cod, for example, keeps for many months. However, when fish is cured to this level it will need a good soaking in several changes of water before use. You can cure most fish for slicing and eating raw – oily fish such as mackerel and bass work exceptionally well.

As I don't need to preserve fish for long periods, I like to give the fish a light curing, so that it can be eaten after a few days. One of the recipes in this section is for curing salmon; it can be kept in the fridge for up to a week. You will see that I use a mixture of salt and sugars (in the form of dark sugar and maple syrup) to balance each other; I also add a few aromatics to the 'cure'. Experiment with the flavours in the cure – dill seeds, coriander seeds, fresh dill, star anise and curry spices will all produce fabulous results.

For more immediate use, I soak monkfish in a very weak brine, made with salt, lemon and fennel seeds, for an hour, then thoroughly dry it before roasting – the results are delicious. If you want to cure a fish to eat straight away, you can immerse it in a mixture of salt, sugar and aromatics, or in citrus juice, just before cooking. Scallops, finely sliced, and marinated in lime juice with a little chopped coriander (cilantro) and chilli (chile), need just a few minutes marinating for a delicious and fresh taste.

This dish was inspired by the excellent Quo Vadis restaurant in Dean Street, London.

lime-cured sea bass with avocado and red onion

SERVES 4 TO START

2 very fresh sea bass fillets, each 200 g/7 oz, skinned, pinboned and cut into chunks

juice of 2 limes

1 mild red chilli (chile), very finely chopped

1 tsp finely chopped fresh mint

1 tbsp very finely chopped celery

1 tbsp very finely chopped red (bell) pepper

1 tbsp very finely chopped green (bell) pepper

1 tbsp very finely chopped red onion

1 avocado, peeled, stoned and cut into chunks roughly the same size as the bass

3 tbsp very best extra virgin olive oil

sea salt and freshly ground black pepper

Simply mix everything together except the seasoning and leave, covered, for 5 minutes. Season to taste, then serve.

AT THE FISHMONGER
Ask your fishmonger to skin and pinbone 2 x 200 g/7 oz
very fresh sea bass fillets.

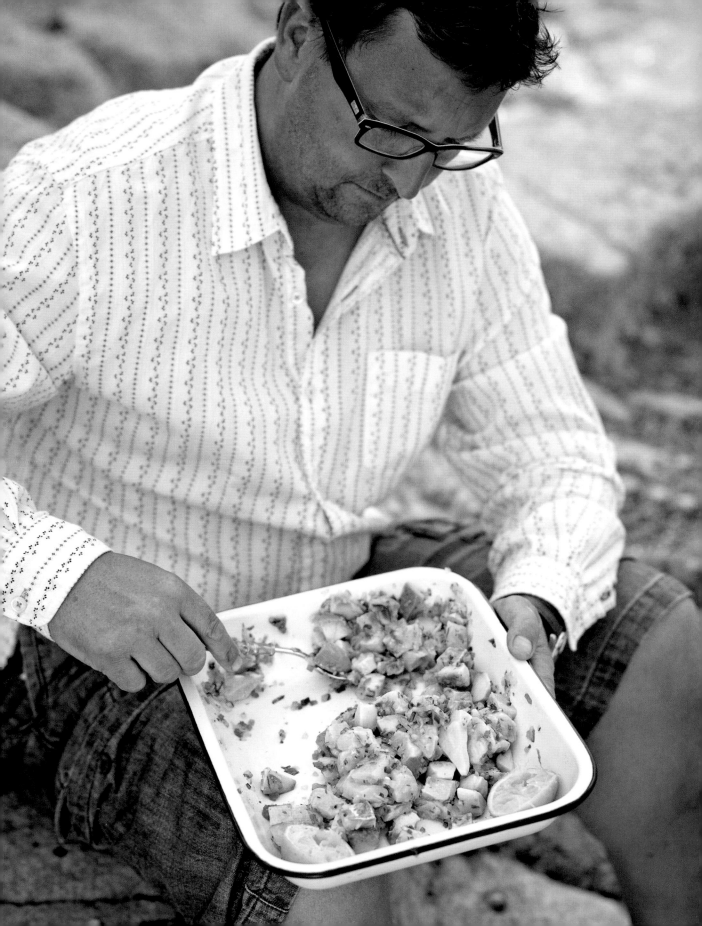

This is a really nice way of using smoked haddock. Buy the best quality you can and look for naturally smoked. The finest I have ever tasted comes from Grimsby, where the old methods have earned them protected status. There are traditional fish smokers there, namely Atkinsons and Alfred Enderby, who in my opinion make the finest smoked haddock in the world.

Jersey potato, smoked haddock, leek and egg salad

SERVES 2

300 ml/10½ fl oz/1¼ cups milk

1 fillet of undyed smoked haddock, 200 g/7 oz, skinned and pinboned

2 tbsp wholegrain mustard

1 tbsp sugar dissolved in 1 tbsp water

6 tbsp mayonnaise (see page 195)

1 small leek, white part only, finely shredded

200 g/7 oz Jersey or early potatoes, washed, boiled and cooled to room temperature

1 tbsp finely chopped fresh chives

sea salt and freshly ground black pepper

2 hard-boiled eggs, whites and yolks separated and finely chopped

Warm the milk over a medium-low heat to a gentle simmer, then add the haddock and poach for 5–6 minutes until moist and cooked. Remove from the milk, flake the fish into a bowl and leave until just warm. Discard the milk.

Mix the mustard with the sugar, then stir into the mayonnaise.

Place the leek, potatoes and mayonnaise in a bowl and stir, then fold in the fish and chives and season. Sprinkle with the chopped egg and serve.

AT THE FISHMONGER
Ask your fishmonger to skin and pinbone a 200 g/7 oz undyed smoked haddock fillet.

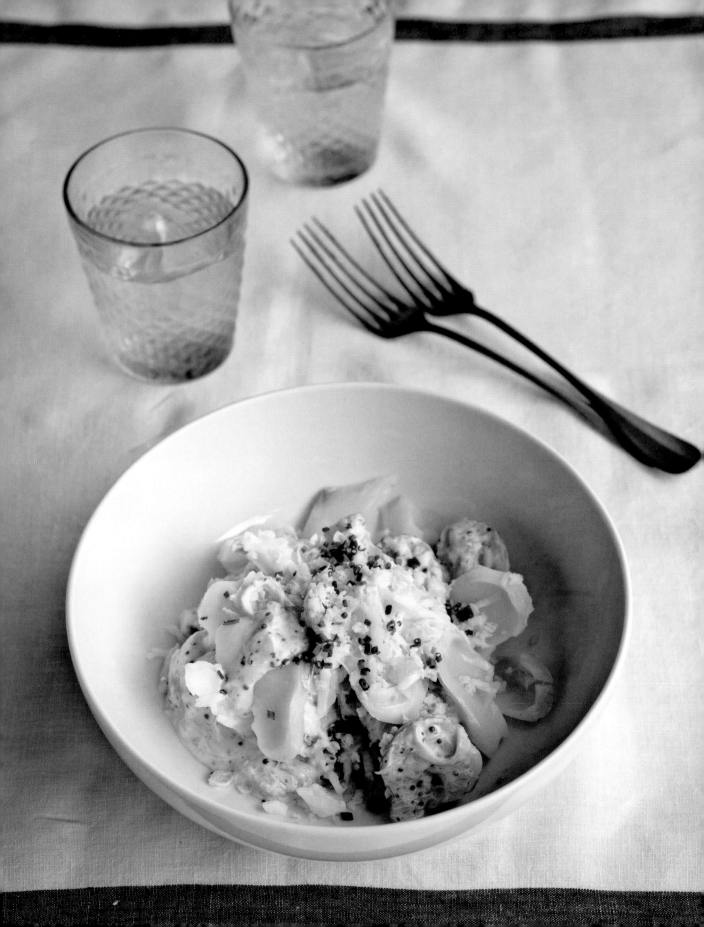

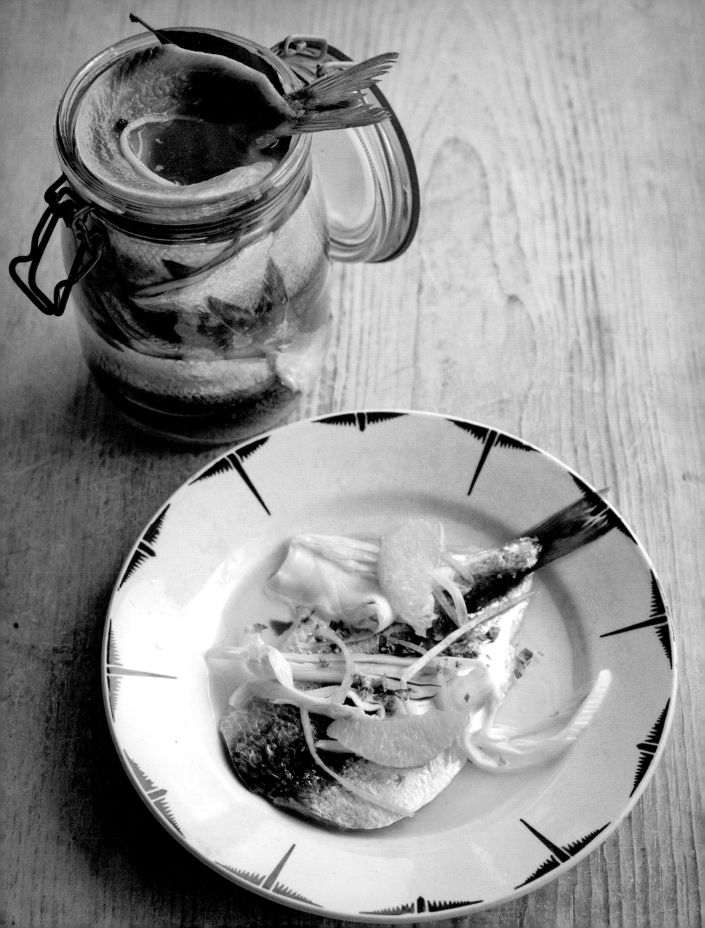

I see a lot of herring here in the bay as early as May. It's a very underrated fish, but is deliciously oily and ideal for curing. Orange and fennel are a perfect foil for each other, but try other fruits such as pink grapefruit, pomegranate or a good lemon; they all work fine. This is worth making in large quantities since the herring keep well in the fridge and with a little salad and some bread they make a fine lunch.

cured herring with orange and fennel

SERVES 12

150 g/5½ oz/¾ cup sea salt

50 g/2 oz/¼ cup caster (superfine) sugar

12 herring fillets, tail on, pinboned

For the pickle

1 fennel bulb, thinly sliced lengthways

400 ml/14 fl oz/1¾ cups white wine vinegar

200 g/7 oz/1 cup caster (superfine) sugar

2 bay leaves

1 star anise

2 cloves

1 tsp black peppercorns

shredded peel of 1 orange

To serve

2 oranges, broken into segments

small handful of fresh flat-leaf parsley, finely chopped

small handful of fresh mint, finely chopped

good olive oil

To make the pickle, put all the ingredients into a saucepan over a medium-high heat and bring to the boil, then take off the heat and leave to cool completely. The flavour should be sweet and sour, as the sugar will have taken the edge off the vinegar.

Mix the salt and sugar together. Dry the herring fillets and lay them, flesh side up, as a single layer in a dish, then sprinkle over the salt and sugar mixture, cover, and leave to cure in the fridge for 3–4 hours. Wash off the salt and sugar and dry with kitchen paper.

Place the fillets in a sterilized jar or non-metallic dish, then pour the pickle mixture over and cover. Leave in the fridge for a day or two (they can be eaten straight away but the flavour improves with time).

Serve each fillet with some of the fennel, orange segments, a sprinkling of parsley and mint and a drizzle of your best olive oil.

AT THE FISHMONGER
Ask your fishmonger to fillet and pinbone 6 herring.

You will need to buy a frozen octopus from the Atlantic for this. They come ready to cook and weigh about 1.5 kg/3 lb 5 oz each. This is worth making for a large table of people. My friend and fellow chef Mark Hix and I cooked it in Portugal on our annual trip to blend our wine, 'Tonnix', and great with the wine it was too!

octopus, potato, caper and oregano salad

SERVES 4

1 frozen octopus, about
1.5 kg/3 lb 5oz, thawed

10 small waxy potatoes, peeled

2 celery sticks (stalks), finely sliced,
plus a few leaves

1 tbsp finely chopped fresh flat-leaf
parsley

For the dressing
pinch of dried oregano flowers, from
the branch if possible

1 tbsp good red wine vinegar

small handful of rinsed capers

1 small red onion, finely sliced

1 small dried chilli (chile)

3–4 tbsp good extra virgin olive oil

Simmer the octopus in a large pan of water for about 1 hour until tender; test it with a knife – there should be little resistance. Leave it to cool in the water.

Meanwhile, make the dressing. Add the oregano flowers to the vinegar in a bowl and soak for 20 minutes. Add the capers and onion, crumble in the chilli and stir in the olive oil.

Cook the potatoes in lightly salted boiling water for 10 minutes, or until tender, then slice them.

Remove the octopus from the water and slice into chunks. Add the potatoes, celery and dressing and turn to coat. Serve on a large platter sprinkled with parsley and celery leaves.

celery with bottarga from Sardinia

SERVES 2

Bottarga is the dried, salted and cured eggs from grey mullet or tuna. Cut **3 sticks of celery** very finely and finely chop the leaves. Grate 1 tsp **grey mullet bottarga** into **the juice of 1 lemon** and leave it to dissolve for a few minutes. Whisk in **3 tbsp olive oil**, **1 tsp** finely chopped **parsley**, **sea salt** and **freshly ground black pepper**. Toss with the celery and leaves and then shave more bottarga liberally over the top.

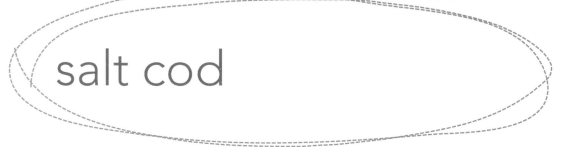

salt cod

Salt cod comes in many different cuts and qualities. Salting was originally a method of preserving cod for transportation or if there was a glut. Salted cod is now highly regarded.

Cod heads and small fillets are salted and dried until hard, and in Norway strips of these are eaten as a snack with the traditional spice-flavoured alcoholic drink, aquavit. At the other end of the scale, I have seen huge fish filleted and the loins salted to end up in Europe's finest markets at a very hefty price.

Different cuts of salt cod are used in different ways – heads, fins and small fillets are used in stews, while fillets from medium fish may end up as *brandade*, a purée with olive oil and garlic, popular in the south of France, or baked with any number of flavours. The larger fillets will be reserved for the finest salads and eating raw, where the texture and flavour are paramount. I have found it easy and economical to salt my own cod. My advice is that where a recipe calls for salt cod, you buy a large thick fillet and do it yourself.

For instructions on how to salt cod, see steps 1–3 overleaf.

This is a good combination of flavours. I like to make my own salt cod by just covering a nice thick loin in rock salt for a few days and then soaking it for at least one day before cooking. It firms it up well for this salad and gives it that lovely savoury note of salted cod.

salad of salted cod, orange, fennel and pomegranate

SERVES 4

300 g/10½ oz piece of cod loin
2 handfuls of rock salt
1 orange, peeled and cut into segments
1 small fennel bulb, finely shaved
½ red onion, very finely sliced
seeds of ½ pomegranate
fresh coriander (cilantro) leaves to serve

For the dressing
100 ml/3½ fl oz/½ cup orange juice
100 ml/3½ fl oz/½ cup lemon juice
100 ml/3½ fl oz/½ cup grapefruit juice
finely grated zest of ½ orange
25 ml/1 fl oz/scant 2 tbsp raspberry vinegar
50 g/2 oz/¼ cup caster (superfine) sugar
pinch of saffron strands
5 coriander seeds
1 star anise
100 ml/3½ fl oz/½ cup olive oil

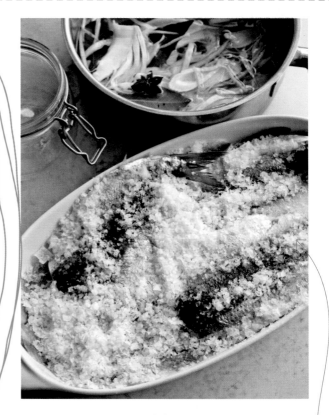

1. Cover the cod in the salt, cover with clingfilm (plastic wrap) and refrigerate for 2 days, each day draining off any liquid in the bottom.

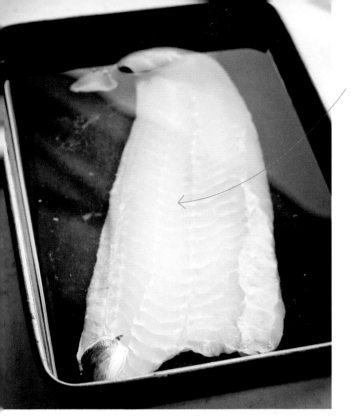

2. Soak the fish in fresh water in the fridge for 1 day, changing the water twice. To see if it is ready, slice off a bit and taste it – it should be firm and slightly salty.

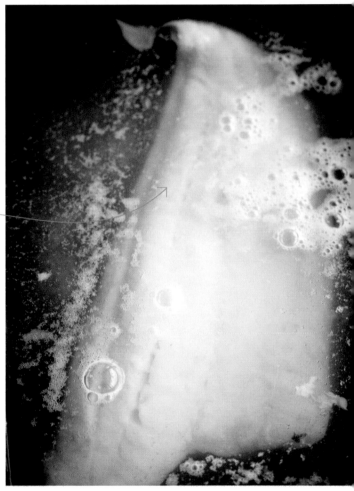

3. Bring a pan of water to the boil. Add the cod and simmer for 1 minute, then take off the heat and leave to cool in the water.

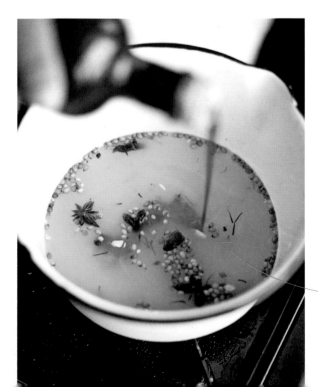

4. Combine all the ingredients for the dressing, except the olive oil, in a saucepan.

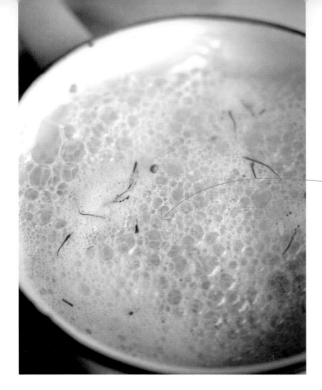

5. Simmer over a medium heat until reduced by half. Remove the spices, then whisk in the olive oil.

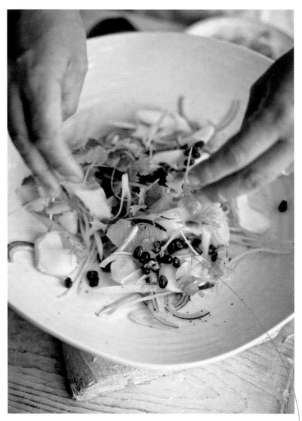

6. Combine the orange segments, fennel and red onion in a bowl, then add the dressing and turn to coat.

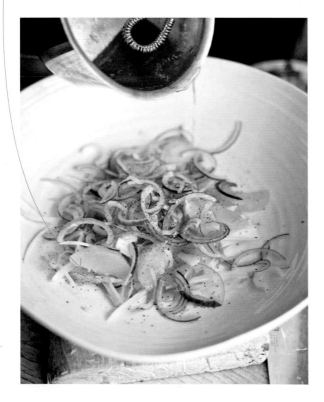

7. Flake in the cod and scatter with the pomegranate seeds and coriander.

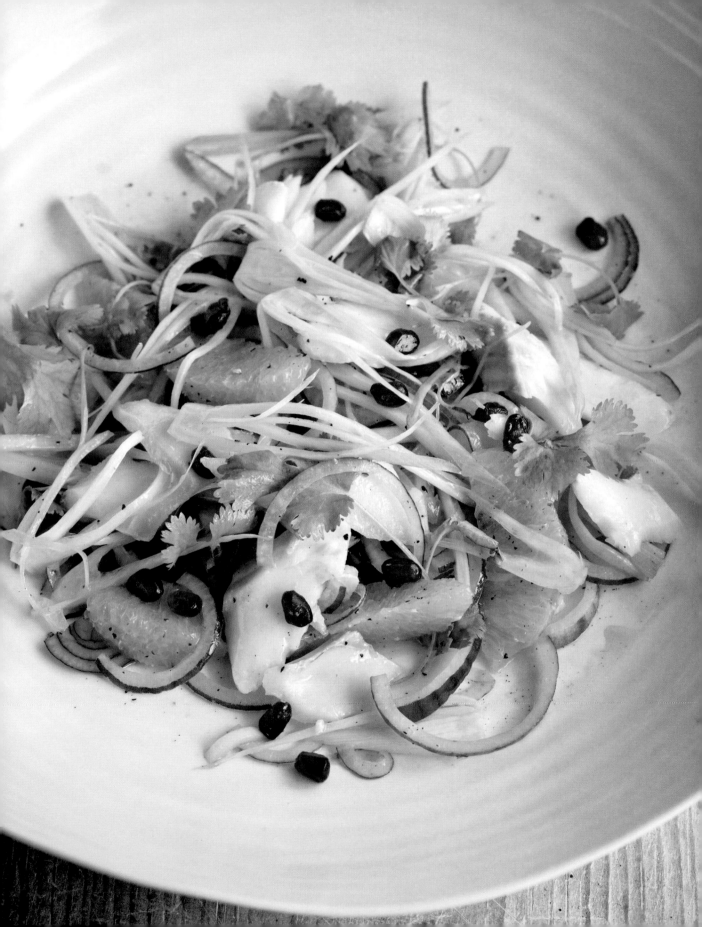

salt cod mayonnaise

SERVES 2

I often make this with the offcuts of salt cod. Soak 150 g/5 oz salt cod in water in the fridge overnight, uncovered, changing the water once or twice. Drain and rinse. Poach the fish in enough milk to cover for 1 minute, then leave to cool in the milk. Drain and shred the fish. Stir the fish into 6 tbsp aioli (see page 196) with some finely chopped curly parsley and a squeeze of lemon. Serve on toast or with some salad leaves. Also try mixing the fish into the anchovy mayonnaise on page 205.

Oily fish such as mackerel and herring work very well filleted and eaten raw with piquant flavours. Sour cream and rye bread are good accompaniments.

mackerel tartare with sour cream and rye bread

SERVES 4

2 very fresh mackerel, each 250 g/9 oz, filleted, pinboned and finely chopped

2 tbsp cornichons (baby gherkins), finely chopped

2 tbsp salted capers, rinsed and finely chopped

1 small red onion, finely chopped

6 tbsp sweet dill and mustard mayonnaise (page 199)

sea salt and freshly ground black pepper

a few drops of Tabasco

watercress, sour cream and rye bread to serve

In a bowl, mix the mackerel, cornichons, capers and red onion with the dill and mustard mayonnaise, then season with sea salt and freshly ground black pepper. Mix in Tabasco to taste. Serve immediately in a pile with the watercress, sour cream and rye bread.

AT THE FISHMONGER
Ask your fishmonger to fillet and pinbone 2 x 250 g/9 oz very fresh mackerel.

I keep roasted peppers in my fridge all the time. Here is a favourite weekday lunch of mine if I'm at home. You could use a poached mackerel or salt cod instead of tuna.

tuna with roasted peppers and capers

SERVES 4

3 red (bell) peppers

250 g/9 oz canned tuna in oil, drained (I like the Spanish producers such as Ortiz, but use your favourite brand)

small handful of salted capers, rinsed

2 tbsp mayonnaise (see page 195)

1 garlic clove, crushed

pinch of smoked paprika

small handful of rocket (arugula) leaves

olive oil

squeeze of lemon

sea salt and freshly ground black pepper

Using a pair of tongs, hold each pepper in a flame on the hob until blackened. (You can put them all on at once and keep moving them about.) Alternatively, preheat the oven to 240°C/475°F/gas mark 9 and cook the peppers for 15–20 minutes.

Put the peppers in a container with a lid, cover and leave to cool. Peel them and discard the skin and seeds. Strain the juices left in the container and reserve. Tear the flesh into strips and lay these on a plate. Drain the tuna and flake it over the peppers, then scatter with capers.

Mix the pepper juices into the mayonnaise to thin it down, then add the garlic and paprika. Drizzle over the salad. Dress the rocket with olive oil and lemon juice and scatter over the salad, then season with salt and freshly ground black pepper and serve.

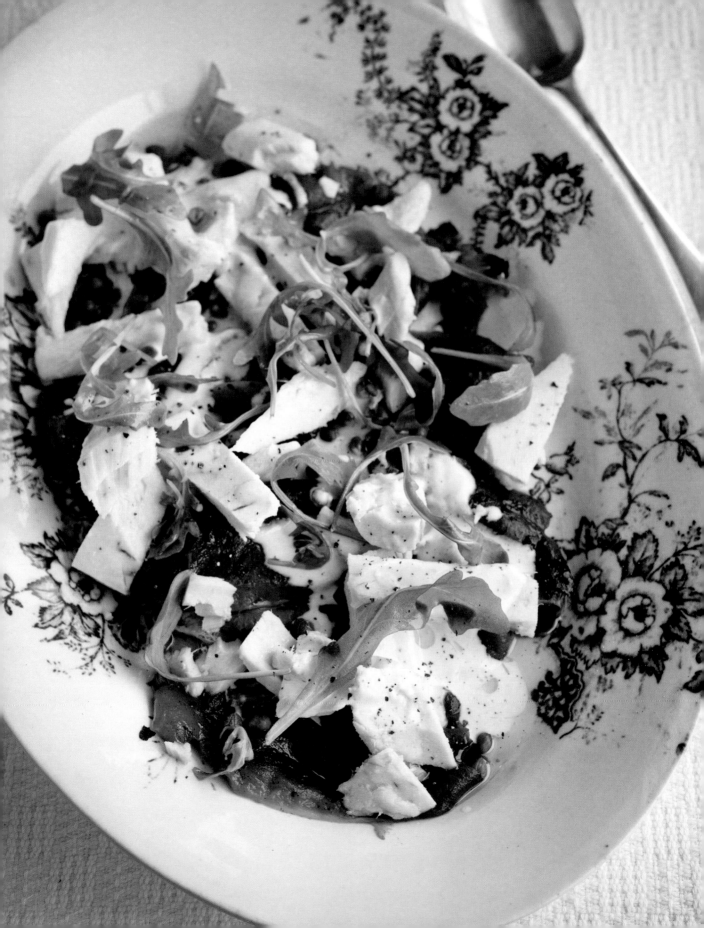

Curing fish is great fun. Salmon cures particularly well and once you have mastered the technique (which is easy), you can play around with spices and flavourings to suit your taste. In essence, a cure removes moisture from the fish, thus preserving it – and this fish can be kept for up to a week. This is best sliced and eaten as it is, with just a few herbs scattered over the top; however, you can roast it too, which gives an interesting flavour.

fennel and maple-cured salmon

MAKES 1 SIDE OF SALMON

1 fillet from a 3–4 kilo salmon, pinboned but skin left on
100 ml/3½ fl oz/½ cup maple syrup
sprinkling of chopped chives to serve
sprinkling of ground fennel seeds to serve
a few pink peppercorns to serve

For the cure
2 tbsp coriander seeds
2 whole star anise
2 tbsp pink peppercorns
2 tbsp fennel seeds
300 g/10½ oz/1 cup rock salt
200 g/7 oz/1 cup soft dark brown sugar

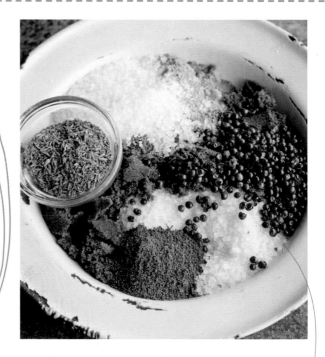

1. Roast the coriander seeds in a hot pan, then grind with the star anise, peppercorns and fennel in a pestle and mortar. Blend in a food processor with the salt and sugar.

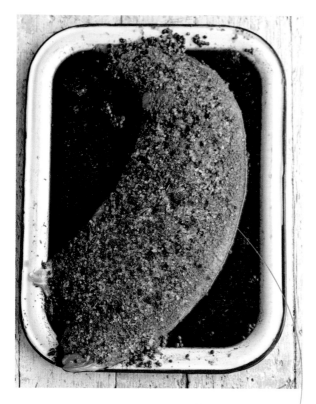

3. Wash off the cure.

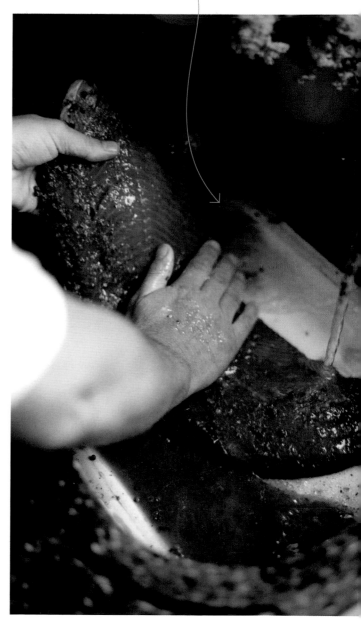

2. Lay the salmon, flesh side up, in a container large enough to hold it flat, then rub it with the maple syrup. Sprinkle the cure over the top. Cover and leave in the fridge overnight. You will notice a lot of liquid appearing – simply mix everything together again, spoon it over the fish and leave for another night in the fridge. Repeat the mixing once more and leave for a further night.

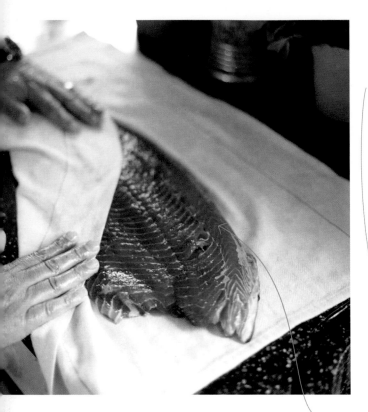

4. Dry the fish thoroughly.

5. The fish is now ready for slicing – cut as smoked salmon, into very thin slices.

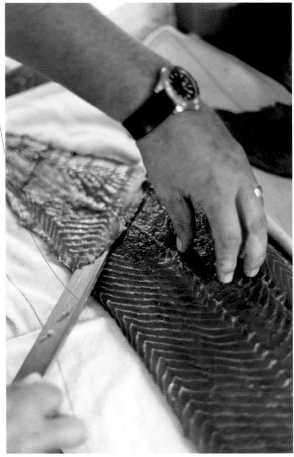

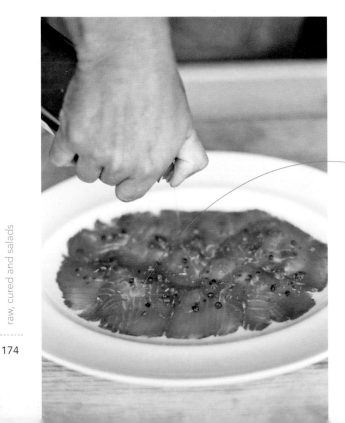

6. Place on a plate and sprinkle with chopped chives, ground fennel seeds and a few pink peppercorns. Drizzle with extra virgin olive oil. The fish can be stored unsliced, wrapped in clingfilm (plastic wrap) in the fridge, for up to a week.

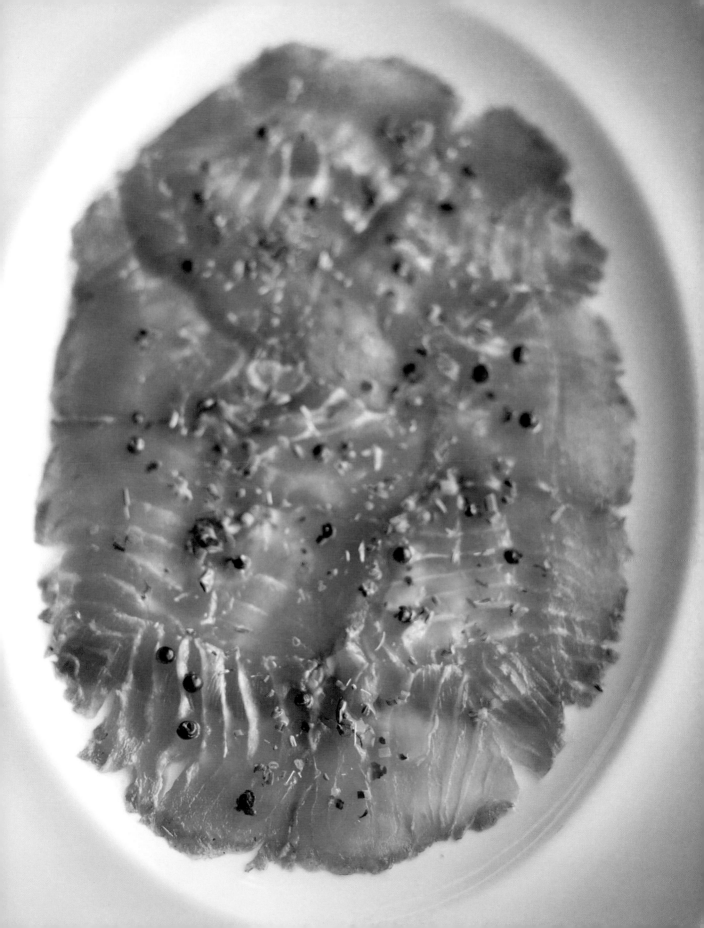

Ginger and mackerel are a nice combination, and this is a great way of preserving a good catch.

pickled mackerel with ginger and lemon

SERVES 4 TO START

4 very fresh mackerel fillets, each about 85 g/3 oz, pinboned

fresh coriander (cilantro) to serve

For the cure
handful of fine salt

handful of caster (superfine) sugar

good pinch of ground cumin

good pinch of ground coriander

good pinch of turmeric

good pinch of ground cinnamon

For the pickle
150 g/5½ oz fresh root ginger, peeled and very finely sliced

300 ml/10 fl oz/1¼ cups white wine vinegar

150 g/5½ oz/¾ cup caster (superfine) sugar

rind of 2 unwaxed lemons, cut into very fine shreds

In a bowl, mix the cure ingredients together. Put the mackerel in a shallow dish, skin side down, in a single layer and cover the flesh side with the cure, then cover and leave in the fridge for 1 hour. Wash and dry the fish.

To make the pickle, mix all the ingredients together in a pan, bring to the boil, then take off the heat and leave to cool.

Place the mackerel in a plastic container. Pour the pickle mixture over it, put the lid on and leave in the fridge for a few days. Serve sprinkled with fresh coriander (cilantro) with good toasted bread.

AT THE FISHMONGER
Ask your fishmonger to fillet and pinbone 2 very fresh mackerel.

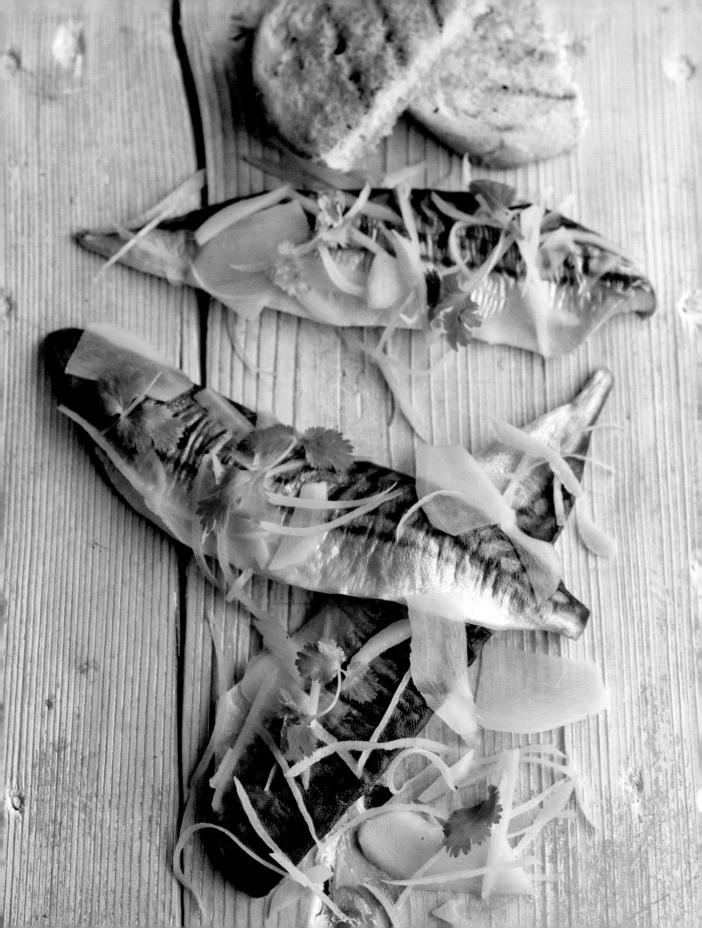

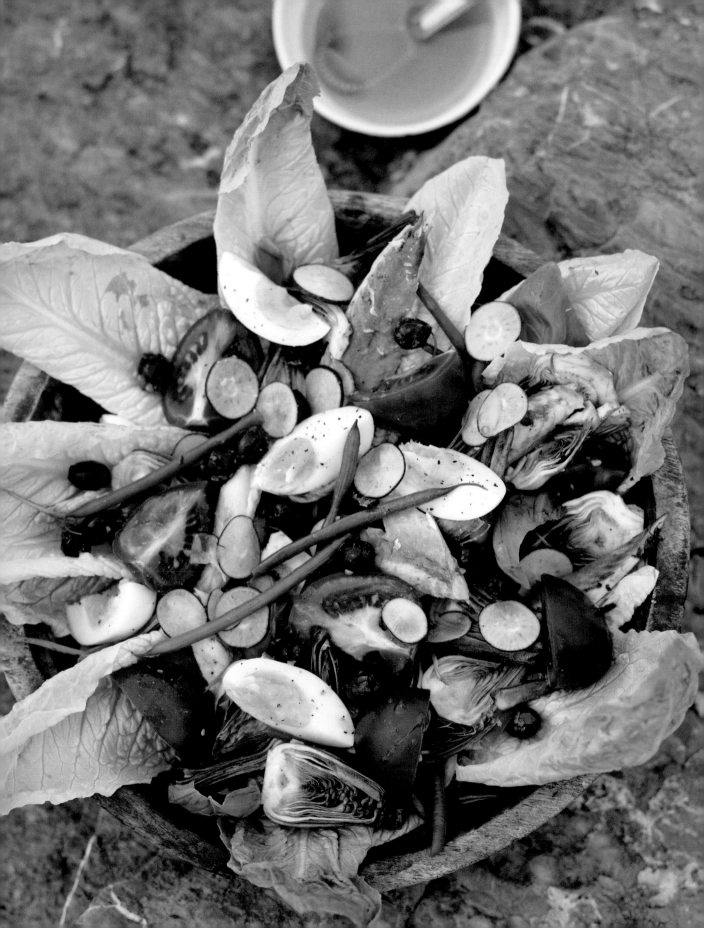

We have so much mackerel in the summer and I am always looking for new ways of using it. I really like the salads from Nice and, with the exception of the olives, we have all the same ingredients locally, so this is our Dartmouth salad!

Dartmouth salad

SERVES 4

4 small mackerel, gutted, heads and tails removed

splash of white wine vinegar

sea salt and freshly ground black pepper

1 bay leaf

100 g/3½ oz green beans, trimmed (I like to use fine runner [string] beans too, but I leave them raw if they are young)

1 lettuce heart, leaves separated

3 very ripe tomatoes, quartered

2 spring onions (scallions), finely sliced

2 small raw artichokes, outer leaves, stem and choke removed and flesh sliced

4 or 5 radishes, finely sliced

6 basil leaves

3 hard-boiled eggs, peeled and quartered

handful of small black olives

For the dressing

3 tbsp good white wine vinegar

9 tbsp good olive oil

6 salted anchovy fillets, ground to a paste

Place the mackerel in a pan with water to cover, the vinegar, a pinch of salt and the bay leaf. Bring to the boil, then take off the heat and leave to cool. Remove the mackerel from the water and flake the fish off the bone into chunks, making sure there are no bones. Blanch the green beans.

To make the dressing, mix the vinegar with the oil and anchovies in a bowl and season well with sea salt and freshly ground black pepper.

Line a bowl with the crisp lettuce leaves, arrange the tomatoes around the edge, then fill the centre with the beans, onions, artichokes, radishes, mackerel and basil. Scatter the eggs and olives over, then dress and toss the salad at the table when everyone is sat down.

AT THE FISHMONGER
Ask your fishmonger to gut and remove the heads and tails from 4 mackerel.

Probably one of my favourite dishes of all time. Really good olive oil is key.

warm salad of seafood and olive oil

SERVES 4

200 g/7 oz each of mussels (scrubbed and wispy beards pulled off), clams and cockles (washed); remove and discard any shells that are broken or open and that do not close when tapped sharply

2 small squid, cleaned and skinned

150 g/5 oz peeled cooked prawns (jumbo shrimp)

For the dressing
3 tbsp olive oil

juice of 1 lemon

1 clove garlic, grated

1 small dried bird's eye chilli, crushed

1 tbsp finely chopped curly parsley

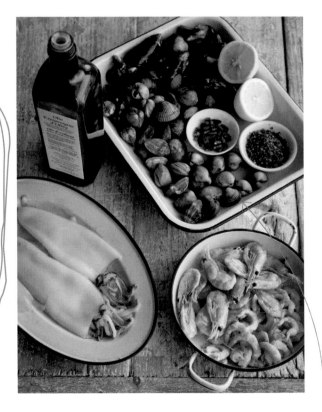

1. Steam the mussels, clams and cockles over 100 ml/ 3½ fl oz water for 3–4 minutes (discard any that remain closed after steaming). Leave them to cool slightly, then remove them from their shells and put in a bowl.

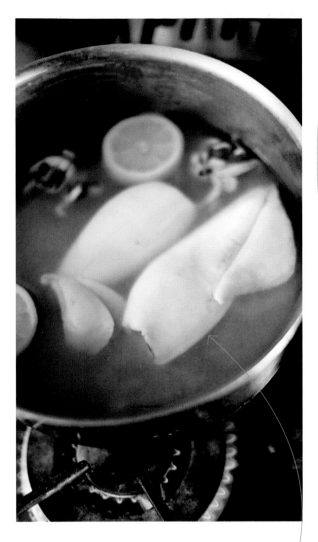

3. Drain the squid and leave to cool, then slice it into thin rings and place it in the bowl with the mussels, clams, cockles and prawns.

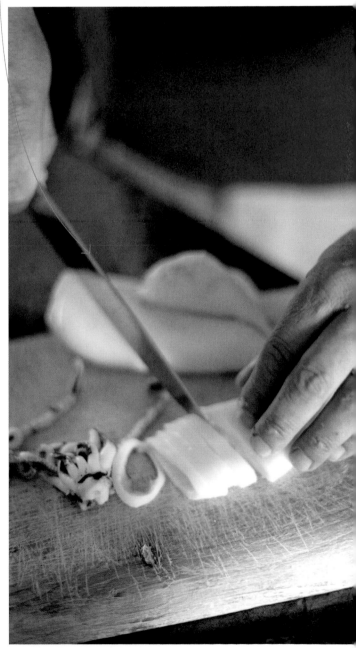

2. Strain the mollusc juices, then add the squid and enough water to cover it. Bring to the boil, then simmer for 4–5 minutes.

4. Combine all the ingredients for the dressing apart from the parsley.

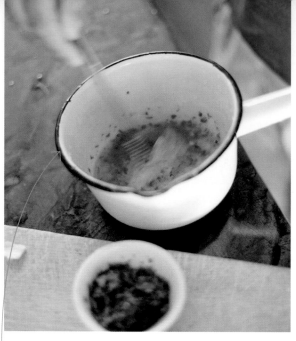

5. Whisk the dressing together, then mix in the parsley.

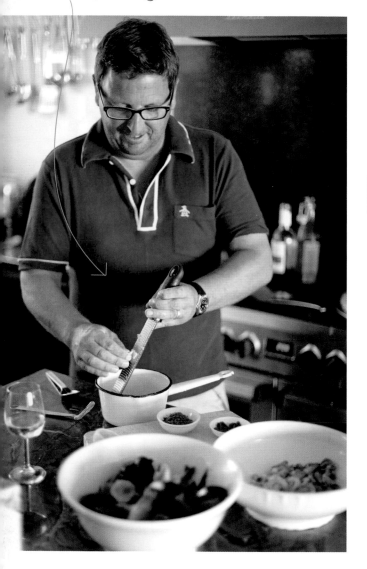

6. Toss the seafood with the dressing and serve warm.

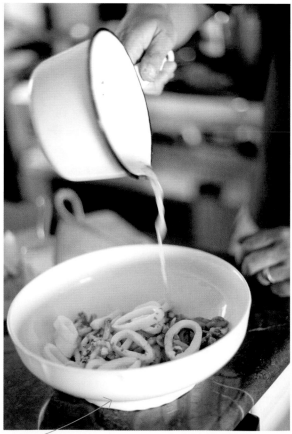

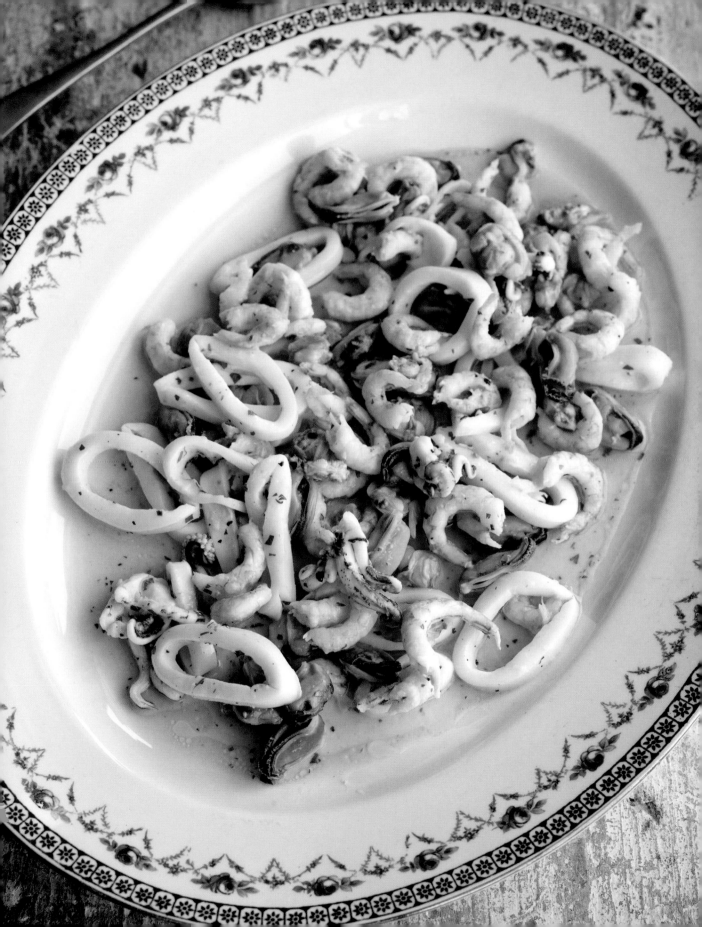

Squid (calamari) is particularly good marinated after being cooked, then eaten at room temperature.

salad of squid with tomatoes and olives

SERVES 4

extra virgin olive oil

2 garlic cloves, finely chopped

350 g/12 oz fresh squid (calamari) with tentacles, cleaned and prepared and cut into thin rings

1 tbsp good white wine vinegar

2 anchovy fillets, pounded to a paste

6 ripe tomatoes, skinned (see page 73) and cut into quarters

small handful of fresh basil leaves

handful of small black olives

Add 1–2 tbsp olive oil to a pan and fry half the garlic over a low heat until just starting to brown. Add the squid and sauté for 2–3 minutes, then take off the heat and transfer to a bowl.

Add the vinegar to the pan and stir to loosen and dissolve any bits on the bottom, then add about 3 tbsp olive oil, stir in the remaining garlic and the anchovies and heat through for about 1 minute.

Toss the squid, tomatoes and most of the basil leaves with the dressing and serve scattered with olives and the remaining basil leaves.

AT THE FISHMONGER
Ask your fishmonger to clean and prepare 350 g/12 oz squid.

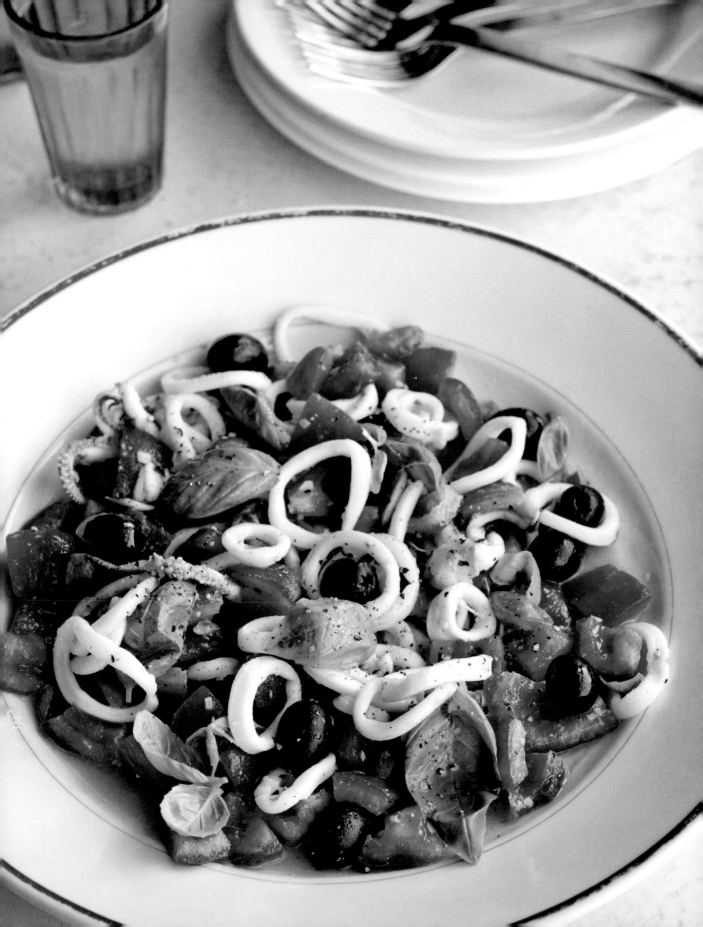

mussel, tomato, garlic and parsley salad

SERVES 4

Prepare and cook 1 kg/2 lb 4 oz mussels (see page 90). Remove from the shells and discard any that remain closed. Preheat the oven to 220°C/425°F/gas mark 7. Wrap a whole head of garlic in foil with a drizzle of olive oil and a sprig of thyme. Place on a baking sheet and roast in the oven for about 20 minutes. Leave to cool. When cooled, squeeze the garlic purée from the skins. Skin, deseed and chop (see page 73) 10 ripe tomatoes of mixed colours and varieties. For the dressing, add 1 tsp Dijon mustard and the juice of 1 lemon to the garlic purée. Gradually whisk in 3 tbsp olive oil until smooth. Season with black pepper and add a handful of finely chopped fresh parsley. Toss the mussels and tomatoes in the dressing and finish with a drizzle of olive oil.

spider crab with lemon and olive oil

SERVES 1

Spider crabs are abundant in UK waters from June to August, but they are mainly exported to Italy and Spain. On the coast, you can buy them either whole or as ready-picked spider crab meat, but if you can't find them, use freshly picked white crab meat from the common brown crab (the meat from the body is best for this). The next most important ingredient is a good peppery extra virgin olive oil. Mix the juice of ½ lemon and 2 tbsp olive oil with 85 g/3 oz cooked white crab meat until the crab is lightly and evenly dressed. Taste and season lightly if needed. Line the top shell of the crab with a few lettuce leaves, then top with the crab mixture and serve.

crab on toast

SERVES 1

A slice of hot **toast**, or even bread, lightly **buttered** and spread with **cooked brown and white crab meat** is a wonderful thing. This is not really a recipe, more a reminder of something special. The following pages give a few other versions of 'crab on toast' that are equally as good.

crab with sherry on toast

SERVES 1

Mix **1 tbsp cooked brown crab meat** with **2 tbsp sherry and caper mayonnaise** on page 207 until loosely bound. Fold in **4 tbsp cooked white crab meat**, then season and serve on toast. The cocktail sauce on page 200 is also very good with cooked white crab meat folded in.

crab with lime, chilli and coriander on toast

SERVES 1

Dress 4 tbsp cooked white crab meat with the juice of 1 lime juice, 1 small finely chopped red chilli (chile) and 1 tbsp finely chopped fresh coriander (cilantro), season with fish sauce to taste and serve on toast.

crab with tarragon and tomato

SERVES 6

A very simple way to enjoy crab, perfect for the summer. Pierce **6 ripe tomatoes** and put in just-boiled water for 2 minutes, then remove, cool and skin them. Cut off the tops, then scoop out the insides and discard. Mix **12 tbsp fresh cooked white crab meat** with **3 tbsp cooked brown crab meat**, add **1 tbsp finely chopped fresh tarragon, 1 tbsp mayonnaise** (see page 195) and **a squeeze of lemon** and mix together well. Stuff each tomato, leaving crab overflowing from the top. Drizzle with **a little olive oil** and scatter **a few basil leaves** over the crab.

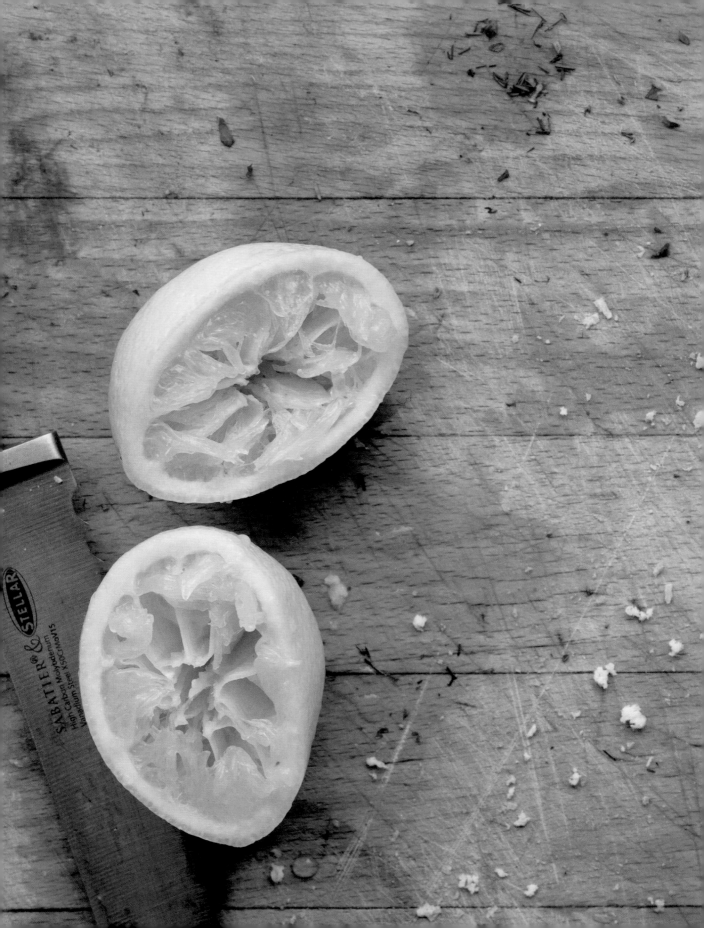

mayonnaise and other basics

mayonnaise and variations

Mayonnaise is a good basic sauce and in various guises is excellent with all seafood, whether poached, grilled, fried or roasted. I find it easy to knock up a batch of basic mayonnaise at the beginning of the week and then make variations as I need them.

You can also use mayonnaise to thicken sauces and soups by whisking a little of the warm cooking liquid into a small amount of mayonnaise, then stirring it into the soup, broth or sauce. It adds a nice creamy richness and is the technique used to make the famous French fish stew *bourride*.

mayonnaise

SERVES 6

Place **3 medium egg yolks, 1 tbsp mustard powder** or Dijon mustard and **2 tbsp white wine vinegar** in a bowl and whisk together. Slowly drizzle in **vegetable oil**, whisking all the time. Keep adding until you have a thick creamy mayonnaise. Season with **fine salt and white pepper**, then taste and add more mustard or vinegar to get the flavour you like. Finish by whisking in **1 tbsp good olive oil**.

herb cream mayonnaise

SERVES 4

Add ½ tbsp each of chopped fresh chervil, basil, chives and tarragon to 8 tbsp mayonnaise (see page 195), then gently fold in the same quantity of whipped cream to lighten it. Serve straight away with poached fish, lobster or crab.

aioli

SERVES 4

Crush 2–3 garlic cloves in a pestle and mortar with a little sea salt until you have a fine paste. Stir this into 6 tbsp mayonnaise (see page 195) and leave, covered in the fridge, for an hour or two before using. For variations, you can stir finely chopped curly parsley, chilli, saffron or lemon through. Serve with fried fish.

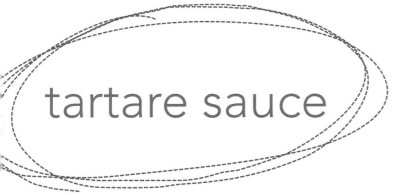

tartare sauce

SERVES 4

Stir 1 tbsp each of finely chopped shallots, tarragon, parsley, capers and cornichons (baby gerkins) into 6 tbsp mayonnaise (see page 195). Serve with fried, grilled or roasted fish.

horseradish mayonnaise

SERVES 4

Stir 1 tbsp horseradish, 1 tbsp Dijon mustard and 1 tbsp finely chopped parsley into 6 tbsp mayonnaise (see page 195). Serve with smoked eel, salmon or trout, or with grilled halibut or other grilled meaty fish.

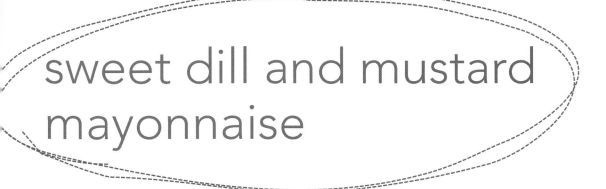

sweet dill and mustard mayonnaise

SERVES 4

Dissolve 1 tbsp caster (superfine) sugar in 2 tbsp white wine vinegar. Mix into 6 tbsp mayonnaise (see page 195) with 2 tbsp Dijon mustard, or to taste. Finish with lots of finely chopped fresh dill. Serve with cured fish and smoked salmon.

cocktail sauce

Stir 25 ml/1 fl oz whisky, dry sherry or brandy, 2 tbsp tomato ketchup and a few drops of Tabasco or pinch of cayenne into 8 tbsp mayonnaise (see page 195). Serve with prawns, crab or lobster.

mayonnaise and other basics

coriander and red chilli aioli

SERVES 4

Peel and deseed **2 ripe tomatoes** (see page 73). Cook down in a pan over a low heat until thickened and the juices are concentrated – about 5–10 minutes. Push through a small sieve, then mix into **8 tbsp aioli** (see page 196) with **lots of chopped fresh coriander (cilantro)** and **2 finely chopped and deseeded red chillies (chiles).** Serve with grilled or roasted fish.

saffron mayonnaise

SERVES 4

Steep a pinch of **saffron strands** in 1 tbsp warm water for a few minutes, then drain and stir into 6–8 tbsp mayonnaise (see page 195) or aioli (see page 196). If you are eating this with a soup or stew, add a little of the liquid to it and **a crumbled dried chilli (chile)** for heat. Serve with soups and stews or grilled fish.

mustard, caper and chervil mayonnaise

SERVES 4

Stir 2 tbsp Dijon mustard, 1 tbsp chopped capers and 2 tbsp mixed fresh chervil, tarragon and chives to taste into 6–8 tbsp mayonnaise (see page 195). Serve with grilled and poached fish; especially good with grilled mackerel, salmon and herring.

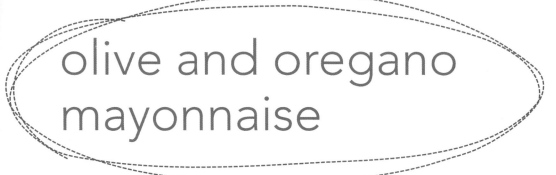

olive and oregano mayonnaise

SERVES 4

Blitz 20 or so pitted black olives in a food processor until very fine, then stir into 6–8 tbsp mayonnaise (see page 195) with a little finely chopped oregano and a squeeze of lemon juice. Use with grilled and roasted fish; especially good with grey and red mullet.

artichoke and anchovy mayonnaise

SERVES 4

Boil **2 artichoke hearts** until tender, then drain and blitz in a food processor. Pass through a small sieve until you have a smooth purée, then mix into **6–8 tbsp aioli** (see page 196) or **mayonnaise** (see page 195). Pound **3 or 4 salted anchovy fillets** to a paste in a pestle and mortar, then stir into the aioli. Simply leave out the artichoke for a very versatile and delicious anchovy mayonnaise. Serve with grilled fish or on roasted vegetables; also works well with poached mackerel.

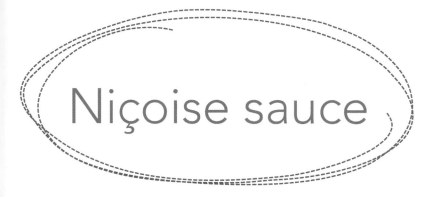

Niçoise sauce

SERVES 2

Skin and deseed **2 ripe tomatoes** (see page 73). Cook down in a pan over a low heat until thickened. Pass through a sieve, then stir into **6–8 tbsp mayonnaise** (see page 195). Add a splash of red wine vinegar, **1 tbsp chopped fresh basil** and **1 tbsp finely chopped black olives**. Serve with grilled mullet or squid, although it's very versatile and works well with any summery fish dish.

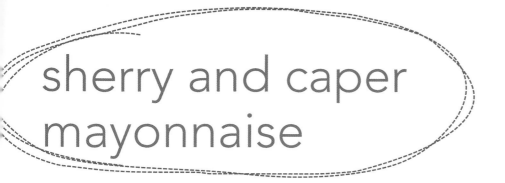

sherry and caper mayonnaise

SERVES 4

Stir **1 tbsp medium sherry, 1 tsp sherry vinegar** and a few **chopped capers** into **6–8 tbsp** mayonnaise (see page 195). Serve with grilled shellfish or grilled oily fish.

This is the backbone of many soups, stews and pasta sauces. It's easy to make and worth cooking in a big batch and then freezing. There is no substitute where it is called for in many recipes.

shellfish stock

**MAKES 4 LITRES/7 PINTS/
4 QUARTS**

3 kg/6 lb 8 oz crab, prawn or lobster
shells

olive oil

1 fennel bulb, finely chopped

2 leeks, finely chopped

2 celery sticks (stalks), finely chopped

2 carrots, finely chopped

4 tbsp tomato purée

1 head of garlic, cut in half
horizontally

handful of parsley stalks

sprig of fresh thyme

2 bay leaves

pinch of saffron strands

1 tbsp black peppercorns

1 tbsp fennel seeds

Preheat the oven to 220°C/425°F/gas mark 7. Place the shells in a roasting pan large enough to take them in one layer. Drizzle olive oil over them, then roast for 15–20 minutes until you can smell them roasting and they are starting to turn lightly golden but are not burning.

Meanwhile, sweat all the vegetables slowly in 4 tbsp olive oil until they are lightly golden. Add the tomato purée and cook for 3–4 minutes, then add the shells and the remaining ingredients. Cover with water and simmer very gently, lid on, for 4–5 hours. Strain, then simmer, lid off, to reduce by half.

It's worth making a batch of this and keeping it in a sterilized jar in the fridge for when you grill fish. Brush the fish with olive oil, or marinate it in a little wine for 10 minutes, before cooking, then lightly sprinkle this mixture over it to give a light coating that will crisp up during cooking.

herb mixture for grilling

1 tbsp dried savory
2 tbsp fennel seeds
2 tbsp dried oregano
2 tbsp crumbled dried bay leaves
2 bird's-eye chillies (chiles)
200 g/7 oz breadcrumbs

Simply blitz together in a food processor and use or store.

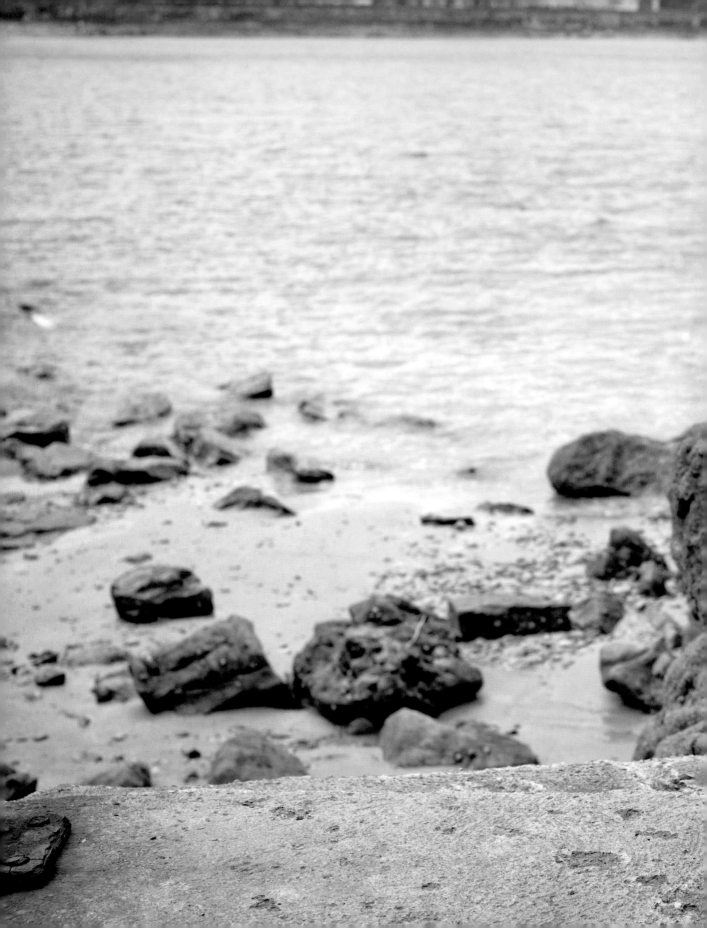

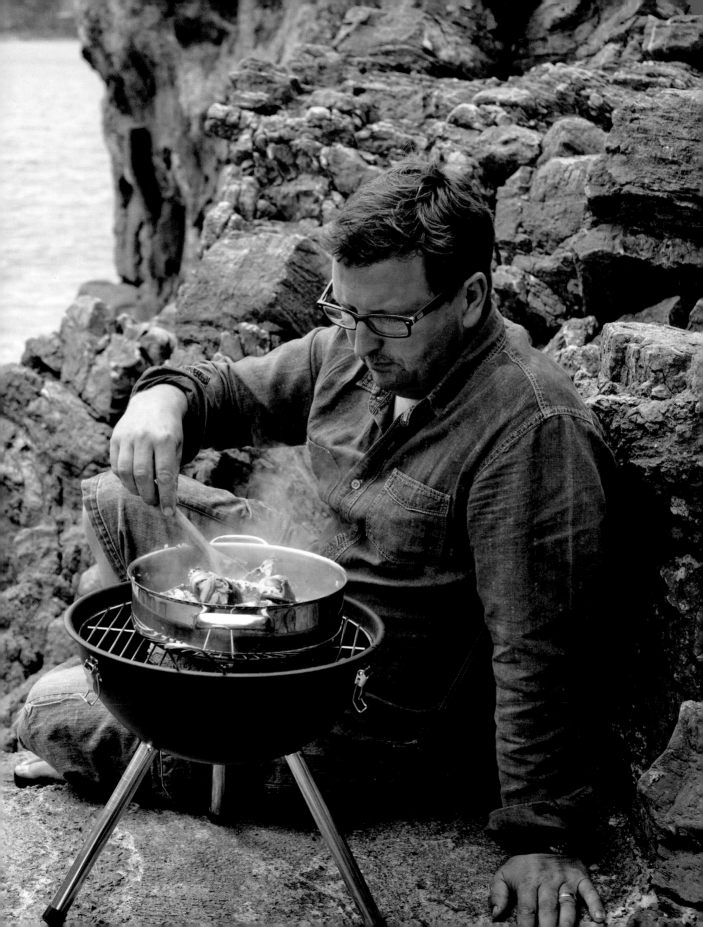

index

A

Adriatic dressing, grilled red mullet with 27
aioli 196
    coriander and red chilli aioli 201
    cuttlefish with summer vegetables, mint and aioli 84
    roast hake with parsley vinaigrette, aioli and boiled
        potatoes 114
    salt cod mayonnaise 168
'al cartoccio' 138
    brill cooked 'al cartoccio' with leeks
        and Riesling 139
anchovy
    anchovy sauce 53
    artichoke and anchovy mayonnaise 205
    pollack with sage, anchovy and greens 115
    red mullet soup 74
    red mullet with anchovy and sage 64, *65*
    salsa Milanese 57
artichoke
    artichoke, garlic and anchovy mayonnaise 205
    cuttlefish with summer vegetables, mint and aioli 84
    Niçoise dressing 54
avocado, lime-cured sea bass with red onion
    and 154, *155*

B

bags, cooking in 138
baked rice with crab and sherry 136
balsamic, roast shellfish with tarragon and *130*, 131
barbecue grill 16–17
barbecue sauce, grilled octopus with 35
basil
    grilled mackerel with lemon, ginger and basil 31
    ray with herbs and capers *104*, 105
    salsa Milanese 57
    sea bass with peperonata and basil *28*, 29
bass *see* sea bass
bay leaves, mussels with chilli, wine and 90, *91*
bottarga: celery with bottarga from Sardinia 161
'bouillabaisse' style, gurnard cooked 121
bread
    crab on toast 188
    crab with sherry on toast 189
    mackerel tartare with sour cream and rye bread 169
breadcrumbs: herb mixture for grilling 209
bream *see* gilt-head bream; sea bream
brill cooked 'al cartoccio' with leeks and Riesling 139
broad beans
    cuttlefish with summer vegetables, mint and aioli 84
    shellfish stew with broad beans and savory 94, *95*
broccoli: pollack with sage, anchovy and greens 115
bucatini with sardines, chard and wild fennel 75
butter
    grilled sole with tarragon butter *22*, 23
    roasted scallops with thyme and coral butter 134, *135*
    steamed lobster with herb butter sauce *88*, 89

C

Café Belaer, Menorca 86
calderata, slow-cooked lobster 132
capers
    grey mullet with dill and capers 110, *111*
    gurnard with onions and capers in agrodolce 122, *123*
    monkfish, caper and olive stew 73
    mustard, caper and chervil mayonnaise 203
    octopus, potato, caper and oregano salad 160
    ray with herbs and capers *104*, 105
    salsa Milanese 57
    sardine fritters with caper mayonnaise 76, *77*
    sherry and caper mayonnaise 207

tartare sauce 197

tuna with roasted pepper and capers 170, *171*

celeriac, monkfish steaks with brown shrimps
and *116*, 117

celery

celery with bottarga from Sardinia 161

gurnard with braised celery and cider 120

chard, bucatini with sardines, wild fennel and 75

chervil: mustard, caper and chervil mayonnaise 203

chorizo: New England-style clam bake 149

cider, gurnard with braised celery and 120

clams

baked spaghetti and clams 146, *147*

clams and peas with sherry with coriander 96

New England-style clam bake 149

roast shellfish with tarragon and balsamic *130*, 131

sailors' clams *92*, 93

sea bass with clams and sherry 70, *71*

shellfish stew with broad beans and savory 94, *95*

warm salad of seafood and olive oil 180–2, *180–3*

cockles

roast shellfish with tarragon and balsamic *130*, 131

shellfish stew with broad beans and savory 94, *95*

warm salad of seafood and olive oil 180-182

cocktail sauce 200

cod

cod with thyme and porcini 145

cod with tomato and ginger 144

see also salt cod

coriander

chilli, mint and coriander yogurt sauce 56

clams and peas with sherry with coriander 96

coriander and red chilli aioli 201

crab with lime, chilli and coriander 190

grilled red mullet with cucumber and coriander 26

crab

baked rice with crab and sherry 136

crab on toast 188

crab with lime, chilli and coriander on toast 190

crab with sherry on toast 189

crab with tarragon and tomato 191

grilled spider crab as cooked in Spain 48, *49*

spider crab with lemon and olive oil 187

cucumber

grilled red mullet with cucumber and coriander 26

poached salmon with cucumber and dill
mayonnaise 72

cured herring with orange and fennel *158*, 159

curing fish 152–3

cuttlefish

cuttlefish with John Susman's nam jim sauce
38–40, *39–41*

cuttlefish with summer vegetables, mint and aioli 84

spaghetti with cuttlefish and ink sauce 82, *83*

D

Dartmouth salad *178*, 179

dill

grey mullet with dill and capers 110, *111*

poached salmon with cucumber and dill
mayonnaise 72

sweet dill and mustard mayonnaise 199

dressings 50

garlic, lemon and parsley dressing 51

Niçoise dressing 54

oregano and chilli dressing 55

E

eggs: Jersey potato, smoked haddock, leek and egg
salad 156, *157*

F

fennel
bucatini with sardines, chard and wild fennel 75
cured herring with orange and fennel *158*, 159
fennel and maple-cured salmon 172–4, *172–5*
gurnard cooked 'bouillabaisse' style 121
salad of salt cod, orange, fennel and
pomegranate 164–6, *164–7*
sea bass with fennel and oregano 141
sea bream with wild fennel and garlic *68*, 69
fennel seeds, grilled sardines with black pepper and 34
fish in salt pastry with lemon, garlic and rosemary 109
fritters, sardine with caper mayonnaise 76, *77*
frozen seafood 9, 10
frying 60–1

G

gilt-head bream: fish in salt pastry with lemon, garlic
and rosemary 109
ginger
braised sea bass in sake and ginger 113
cod with tomato and ginger 144
grilled mackerel with lemon, ginger and basil 31
pickled mackerel with ginger and lemon 176, *177*
grey mullet with dill and capers 110, *111*
grilling 16–19
barbecue grill 16–17
flat grill and grill plates 18
gurnard
grilled gunard with garlic and wine vinegar 25
gurnard baked with potatoes, spinach and white
wine 125
gurnard cooked 'bouillabaisse' style 121
gurnard with braised celery and cider 120
gurnard with onions and capers in agrodolce 122, *123*
gurnard with oysters and leeks 63
gurnard with roasted prawns and Marsala 124
gurnard with sage and pancetta 143

H

hake: roast hake with parsley vinaigrette, aioli and
boiled potatoes 114
herb butter sauce, steamed lobster with *88*, 89
herb cream mayonnaise 196
herb mixture for grilling 209
herring
cured herring with orange and fennel *158*, 159
herring roe pâté 78
Hix, Mark 160
horseradish mayonnaise 198

J

Jersey potato, smoked haddock, leek and egg
salad 156, *157*
John Dory
John Dory with Messina sauce 102, *103*
John Dory with samphire sauce 20, *21*
mixed grill of seafood 42, *43*

L

leeks
brill cooked 'al cartoccio' with leeks and Riesling 139
gurnard with oysters and leeks 63
Jersey potato, smoked haddock, leek and egg
salad 156, *157*
lemon sole: grilled sole with tarragon butter *22*, 23
lime:
crab with lime, chilli and coriander on toast 190
lime-cured sea bass with avocado and red onion 154, *155*
warm salad of seafood and olive oil 180–2, *180–3*

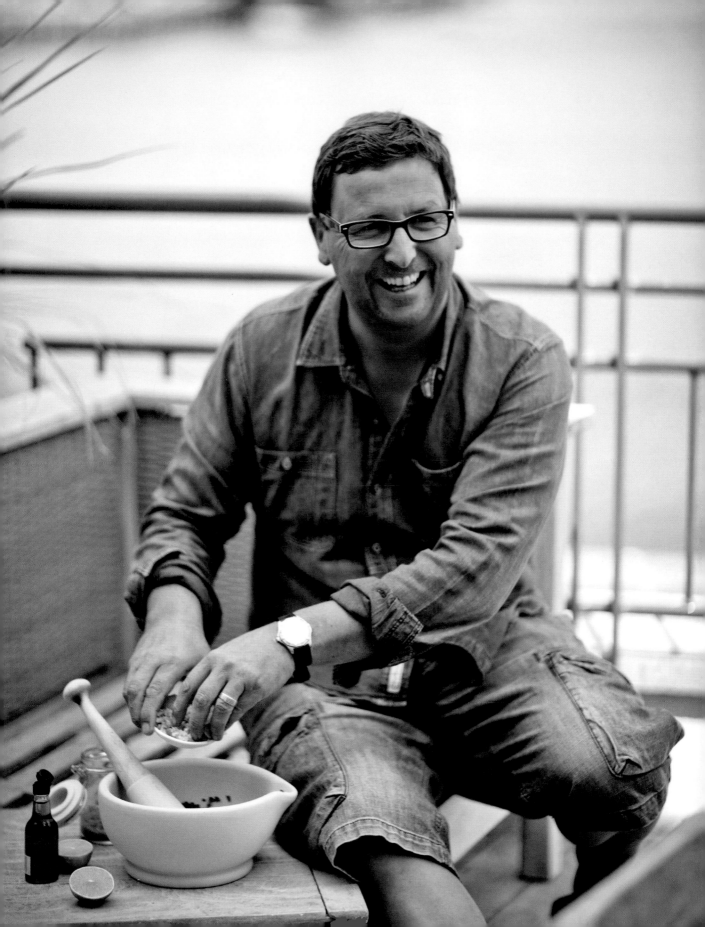

lobster
  braised lobster with sherry and onions 86, *87*
  grilled lobster with chilli and rosemary 44–6, *45–7*
  lobster with herb butter sauce *88*, 89
  mixed grill of seafood 42, *43*
  shellfish stew with broad beans and savory 94, *95*
  slow-cooked lobster caldereta 132

M

mackerel
  baked mackerel with potatoes and thyme *126*, 127
  Dartmouth salad *178*, 179
  grilled mackerel with lemon, ginger and basil 31
  grilled mackerel with spiced salt 32, *33*
  mackerel paste 79
  mackerel tartare with sour cream and rye bread 169
  pickled mackerel with ginger and lemon 176, *177*
maple syrup: fennel and maple-cured salmon 172–4,
  172–5
marrow, pollack with parsley and 142
Marsala, gurnard with roasted prawns and 124
'Mat the clam' 29
Menorca 86
Messina sauce, John Dory with 102, *103*
mint
  chilli, mint and coriander yogurt sauce 56
  cuttlefish with summer vegetables, mint and aioli 84
mixed grill of seafood 42, *43*
monkfish
  mixed grill of seafood 42, *43*
  monkfish as grilled in Romagna 30
  monkfish, caper and olive stew 73
  monkfish steaks with celeriac and brown
    shrimps *116*, 117
  monkfish with sage and roasted garlic 118, *119*
mullet *see* red mullet

mushrooms
  cod with thyme and porcini 145
  plaice with porcini, garlic and parsley 106, *107*
mussels
  mussel, tomato, garlic and parsley salad 186
  mussels with chilli, wine and bay leaves 90, *91*
  New England-style clam bake 149
  roast shellfish with tarragon and balsamic *130*, 131
  roast squid stuffed with mussels, lemon and spinach
    128, *129*
  scallops and mussels 148
  shellfish stew with broad beans and savory 94, *95*
  sole with mussels 108
  warm salad of seafood and olive oil 180–2, *180–3*
mustard
  mustard, caper and chervil mayonnaise 203
  sweet dill and mustard mayonnaise 199

N

nam jim sauce, cuttlefish with 38–40, *39–41*
New England-style clam bake 149
Niçoise dressing 54
Niçoise sauce 206
Norway 10–11
Norwegian Seafood 5

O

octopus
  grilled octopus with barbecue sauce 35
  octopus, potato, caper and oregano salad 160
olive oil, spider crab with lemon and 187
olives
  grilled red mullet with Adriatic dressing 27
  John Dory with Messina sauce 102, *103*
  monkfish, caper and olive stew 73
  Niçoise dressing 54

olive and oregano mayonnaise 204

roast sea bass with potatoes and olives 112

salad of squid with tomato and olives 184, *185*

orange

cured herring with orange and fennel *158*, 159

salad of salt cod, orange, fennel and
pomegranate 164–6, *164–7*

oregano

grilled squid with oregano and chilli *36, 37*

octopus, potato, caper and oregano salad 160

olive and oregano mayonnaise 204

oregano and chilli dressing 55

sea bass with fennel and oregano 141

oysters, gurnard with leeks and 63

P

pancetta, gurnard with sage and 143

'en papillote' 138

parsley

braised razor clams with parsley, sherry
and peas 137

chilli, parsley and roast pepper sauce 52

garlic, lemon, parsley and olive oil dressing 51

mussel, tomato, garlic and parsley salad 186

plaice with porcini, garlic and parsley 106, *107*

pollack with parsley and marrow 142

ray with herbs and capers *104*, 105

roast hake with parsley vinaigrette, aioli and boiled
potatoes 114

roast sea bass with potatoes and olives 112

squid with pearl onions, peas and parsley 85

pasta

baked spaghetti and clams 146, *147*

bucatini with sardines, chard and wild fennel 75

ragù of red mullet with penne *66, 67*

spaghetti with cuttlefish and ink sauce 82, *83*

paste, mackerel 79

pâté, herring roe 78

peas

braised razor clams with parsley, sherry and
peas 137

clams and peas with sherry with coriander 96

cuttlefish with summer vegetables, mint and aioli 84

squid with pearl onions, peas and parsley 85

penne, ragù of red mullet with *66, 67*

pepper

fried squid with chilli-salt and pepper 81

grilled sardines with fennel seed and black pepper 34

peppers

baked rice with crab and sherry 136

chilli, parsley and roast pepper sauce 52

grilled squid with oregano and chilli *36, 37*

sea bass with peperonata and basil *28, 29*

slow-cooked lobster caldereta 132

tuna with roasted pepper and capers 170, *171*

pickled mackerel with ginger and lemon 176, *177*

plaice with porcini, garlic and parsley 106, *107*

pollack

pollack with parsley and marrow 142

pollack with sage, anchovy and greens 115

pomegranate, salad of salted cod, orange, fennel
and 164–6, *164–7*

porcini mushrooms

cod with thyme and porcini 145

plaice with porcini, garlic and parsley 106, *107*

potatoes

baked mackerel with potatoes and thyme *126*, 127

gurnard baked with potatoes, spinach and white
wine 125

gurnard cooked 'bouillabaisse' style 121

Jersey potato, smoked haddock, leek and egg
salad 156, *157*

monkfish steaks with celeriac and brown shrimps *116*, 117

New England-style clam bake 149

octopus, potato, caper and oregano salad 160

roast hake with parsley vinaigrette, aioli and boiled potatoes 114

roast sea bass with potatoes and olives 112

prawns

    gurnard with roasted prawns and Marsala 124

    mixed grill of seafood 42, *43*

    pan-roasted prawns in sticky chilli sauce 97

    roast shellfish with tarragon and balsamic *130*, 131

    shellfish stew with broad beans and savory 94, *95*

    warm salad of seafood and olive oil 180–2, *180–3*

    see also shrimps

Q

Quo Vadis, London 154

R

ragù of red mullet with penne 66, *67*

raw fish, curing 142–3

ray with herbs and capers *104*, 105

razor clams: braised razor clams with parsley, sherry and peas 137

red mullet

    grilled red mullet with Adriatic dressing 27

    grilled red mullet with cucumber and coriander 26

    ragù of red mullet with penne 66, *67*

    red mullet soup 74

    red mullet with anchovy and sage 64, *65*

rice: baked rice with crab and sherry 136

roasting fish 100–1

roe

    celery and bottarga from Sardinia 161

    herring roe pâté 78

rosemary

    fish in salt pastry with lemon, garlic and rosemary 109

    grilled lobster with chilli and rosemary 44–6, *45–7*

    sea bream with roasted garlic, chilli and rosemary 140

rye bread, mackerel tartare with sour cream and 169

S

sage

    gurnard with sage and pancetta 143

    monkfish with sage and roasted garlic 118, *119*

    pollack with sage, anchovy and greens 115

    red mullet with anchovy and sage 64, *65*

sailors' clams 92, *93*

sake, braised sea bass in ginger and 113

salads

    Dartmouth salad *178*, 179

    Jersey potato, smoked haddock, leek and egg salad 156, *157*

    mussel, tomato, garlic and parsley salad 186

    octopus, potato, caper and oregano salad 160

    salad of salt cod, orange, fennel and pomegranate 164–6, *164–7*

    salad of squid with tomato and olives 184, *185*

    warm salad of seafood and olive oil 180–2, *180–3*

salmon

    fennel and maple-cured salmon 172–4, *172–5*

    poached salmon with cucumber and dill mayonnaise 72

salt

    curing fish 142–3

    fried squid with chilli salt and pepper 81

salt cod 162–3

    salad of salt cod, orange, fennel and pomegranate 164–6, *164–7*

    salt cod and onions 133

    salt cod mayonnaise 168

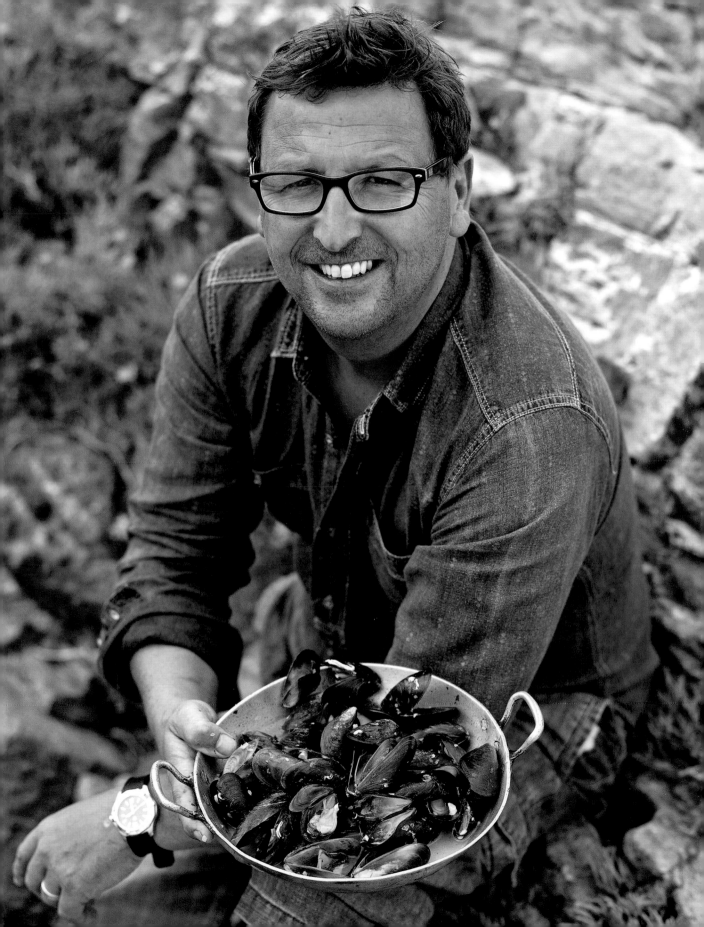

salt pastry, fish in 109

samphire sauce, John Dory with 20, *21*

sardines

    bucatini with sardines, chard and wild fennel 75

    grilled sardines with fennel seed and black pepper 34

    sardine fritters with caper mayonnaise 76, *77*

Sardinia 161

sauces 50

    anchovy sauce 53

    chilli, mint and coriander yogurt sauce 56

    chilli, parsley and roast pepper sauce 52

    cocktail sauce 200

    Niçoise sauce 206

    salsa Milanese 57

    tartare sauce 197

savory, shellfish stew with broad beans and 94, *95*

scallops

    roasted scallops with thyme and coral butter 134, *135*

    scallops and mussels 148

sea bass

    braised sea bass in sake and ginger 113

    lime-cured sea bass with avocado and red onion 154, *155*

    roast sea bass with potatoes and olives 112

    sea bass with clams and sherry 70, *71*

    sea bass with fennel and oregano 141

    sea bass with peperonata and basil *28, 29*

sea bream

    bream with sorrel and cumin 24

    sea bream with roasted garlic, chilli and rosemary 140

    sea bream with wild fennel and garlic 68, *69*

seafood

    mixed grill of seafood 42, *43*

    warm salad of seafood and olive oil 180–2, *180–3*

shellfish

    roast shellfish with tarragon and balsamic *130*, 131

shellfish stew with broad beans and savory 94, *95*

shellfish stock 136, 208

sherry

    baked rice with crab and sherry 136

    braised lobster with sherry and onions 86, *87*

    braised razor clams with parsley, sherry and peas 137

    clams and peas with sherry with coriander 96

    crab with sherry on toast 189

    sea bass with clams and sherry 70, *71*

    sherry and caper mayonnaise 207

shrimps

    monkfish steaks with celeriac and brown shrimps *116, 117*

    see also prawns

Sicily 94, 102, 124

skate *see* ray

smoked haddock: Jersey potato, smoked haddock, leek and egg salad 156, *157*

sole

    grilled sole with tarragon butter 22, 23

    sole fillets as prepared in Venice 62

    sole with mussels 108

sorrel, bream with cumin and 24, *25*

soup

    gurnard cooked 'bouillabaisse' style 121

    red mullet soup 74

sour cream, mackerel tartare with rye bread and 169

spaghetti

    baked spaghetti and clams 146, *147*

    spaghetti with cuttlefish and ink sauce 82, *83*

spider crab

    grilled spider crab as cooked in Spain 48, *49*

    spider crab with lemon and olive oil 187

spinach

    gurnard baked with potatoes, spinach and white wine 125

roast squid stuffed with mussels, lemon and
    spinach 128, *129*

squid
    fried squid with chilli-salt and pepper 81
    grilled squid with oregano and chilli *36, 37*
    mixed grill of seafood 42, *43*
    roast squid stuffed with mussels, lemon and
        spinach 128, *129*
    salad of squid with tomato and olives 184, *185*
    squid with pearl onions, peas and parsley 85
    Vietnamese-style fried squid 80
    warm salad of seafood and olive oil 180–2, *180–3*

stew
    monkfish, caper and olive stew 73
    shellfish stew with broad beans and savory 94, *95*
    slow-cooked lobster caldereta 132

stock, shellfish 136, 208

Susman, John 38

sweet dill and mustard mayonnaise 199

T

tarragon
    crab with tarragon and tomato 191
    grilled sole with tarragon butter *22, 23*
    roast shellfish with tarragon and balsamic *130*, 131

tartare sauce 197

thyme
    baked mackerel with potatoes and thyme *126*, 127
    cod with thyme and porcini 145
    roasted scallops with thyme and coral butter 134, *135*

tiger prawns: pan-roasted prawns in sticky chilli
    sauce 97

toast
    crab on toast 188
    crab with lime, chilli and coriander on toast 190
    crab with sherry on toast 189

tomatoes
    cod with tomato and ginger 144
    coriander and red chilli aioli 201
    crab with tarragon and tomato 191
    grilled octopus with barbecue sauce 35
    John Dory with Messina sauce 102, *103*
    monkfish, caper and olive stew 73
    mussel, tomato, garlic and parsley salad 186
    Niçoise dressing 54
    Niçoise sauce 206
    ragù of red mullet with penne 66, *67*
    red mullet soup 74
    salad of squid with tomato and olives 184, *185*
    sea bass with peperonata and basil *28, 29*

Tsuyu base: braised sea bass in sake and ginger 113

tuna with roasted pepper and capers 170, *171*

V

Venice, sole fillets as prepared in 62

Vietnamese-style fried squid 80

W

wine
    brill cooked 'al cartoccio' with leeks and Riesling 139
    gurnard baked with potatoes, spinach and white
        wine 125
    gurnard with roasted prawns and marsala 124
    John Dory with Messina sauce 102, *103*
    mussels with chilli, wine and bay leaves 90, *91*
    roast sea bass with potatoes and olives 112

Y

yogurt: chilli, mint and coriander yogurt sauce 56

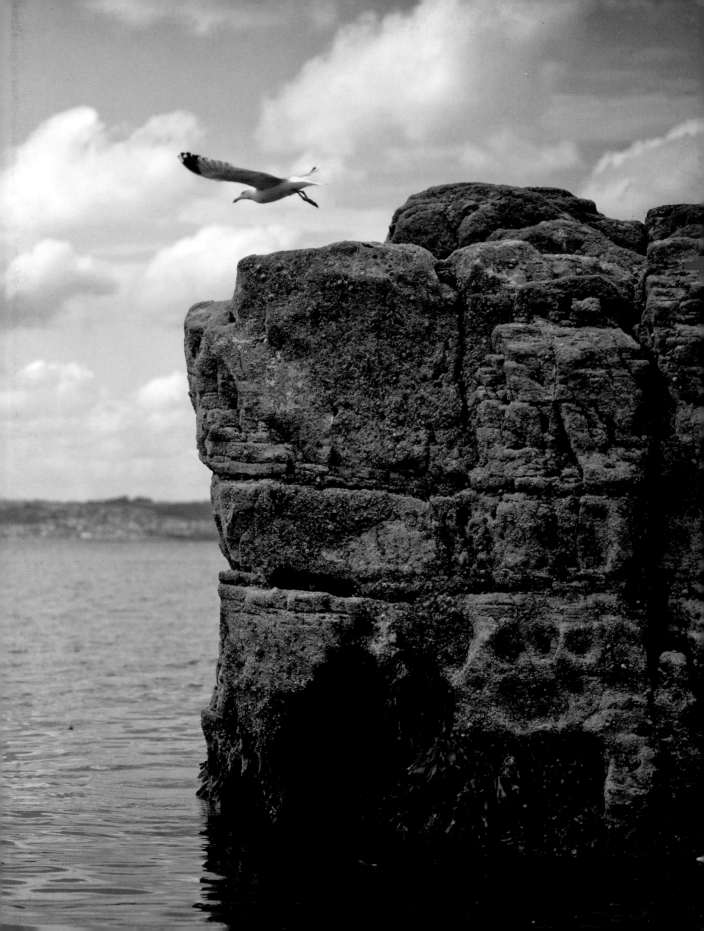

acknowledgements

Gratitude is due to many people for the help they have given me in writing this book. Firstly and mostly, they go to my great pal and partner at The Seahorse, Mat 'The clam' Prowse: you're a legend as always mate, I can't thank you enough for all you do.

Big thanks also to the rest of the team at The Seahorse: Jake 'Elron' Bridgewood, James C, Peter, Maris and the new guy Ben Tonks! It's great cooking with you all.

Thanks also to my amazing front of house team: Nathan 'Turkish' Doyle, Mel B, Ainsley and Sarah Jane, and all the team at RockFish who do a fabulous job every day sprinkling the magic. Big thanks to my assistant Laura, without whom I would not have finished this or any other book!

Thanks also to my agent Annie, and to Becca Spry and all the team at Anova – it's great working with you all.

Wynne, Jim, David and Richard – thanks for all your support in getting us to where we are, you've been truly amazing.

Lastly, thanks to my lovely wife and top mate Pen, who allows me to be me.